Wittlinger

Textbook of Dr. Vodder's
Manual Lymph Drainage

Volume 1: Basic Course

Textbook of Dr. Vodder's Manual Lymph Drainage

Volume 1: Basic Course

Guenther Wittlinger
Former Director
Dr. Vodder School
Walchsee, Germany

Hildegard Wittlinger
Former Director
Dr. Vodder School
Walchsee, Germany

Seventh edition

With 18 illustrations and 2 portraits

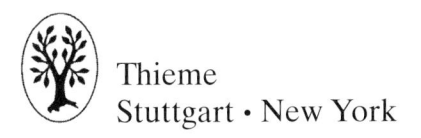

Thieme
Stuttgart · New York

Library of Congress Cataloging-in-Publications Data

This book is an unchanged reprint of the 6th revised English edition published and copyrighted 1998 by Karl F. Haug Verlag, Heidelberg.

Translation revised and edited by Robert H. Harris H.N.D (App. Biol., UK)

1st–12th German edition 1978–1998
Karl F. Haug Verlag, D-Heidelberg
1st–5th English edition
Editions Haug International, B-Brussels

© 2004 Georg Thieme Verlag,
Rüdigerstrasse 14, 70469 Stuttgart, Germany
http://www.thieme.de
Thieme New York, 333 Seventh Avenue, New York, NY 10001 USA
http://www.thieme.com

Typesetting by Datascan GmbH, D-67346 Speyer
Printed in Germany by Druckhaus Beltz, D-69502 Hemsbach

ISBN 3-13-137377-6 (GTV)
ISBN 1-58890-234-X (NTY)

Important note: Medicine is an ever-changing science undergoing continual development. Research and clinical experience are continually expanding our knowledge, in particular our knowledge of proper treatment and drug therapy. Insofar as this book mentions any dosage or application, readers may rest assured that the authors, editors, and publishers have made every effort to ensure that such references are in accordance with **the state of knowledge at the time of production of the book.**
Nevertheless, this does not involve, imply, or express any guarantee or responsibility on the part of the publishers in respect to any dosage instructions and forms of applications stated in the book. **Every user is requested to examine carefully** the manufacturers' leaflets accompanying each drug and to check, if necessary in consultation with a physician or specialist, whether the dosage schedules mentioned therein or the contraindications stated by the manufacturers differ from the statements made in the present book. Such examination is particularly important with drugs that are either rarely used or have been newly released on the market. Every dosage schedule or every form of application used is entirely at the user's own risk and responsibility. The authors and publishers request every user to report to the publishers any discrepancies or inaccuracies noticed.

Some of the product names, patents, and registered designs referred to in this book are in fact registered trademarks or proprietary names even though specific reference to this fact is not always made in the text. Therefore, the appearance of a name without designation as proprietary is not to be construed as a representation by the publisher that it is in the publics domain.

This book, including all parts thereof, is legally protected by copyright. Any use, exploitation, or commercialization outside the narrow limits set by copyright legislation, without the publisher's consent, is illegal and liable to prosecution. This applies in particular to photostat reproduction, copying, mimeographing, preparation of microfilms, and electronic data processing and storage.

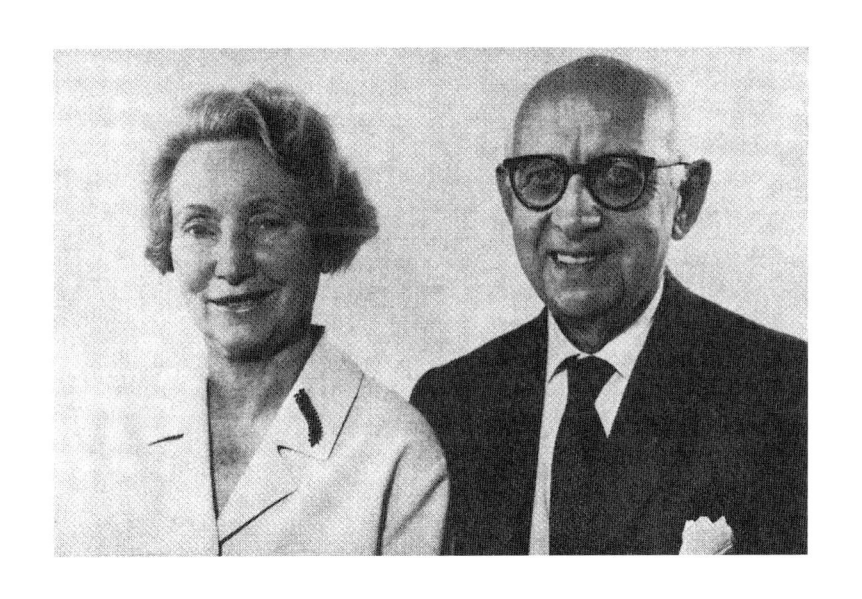

Dedicated to our esteemed teachers
Estrid Vodder † and Emil Vodder †

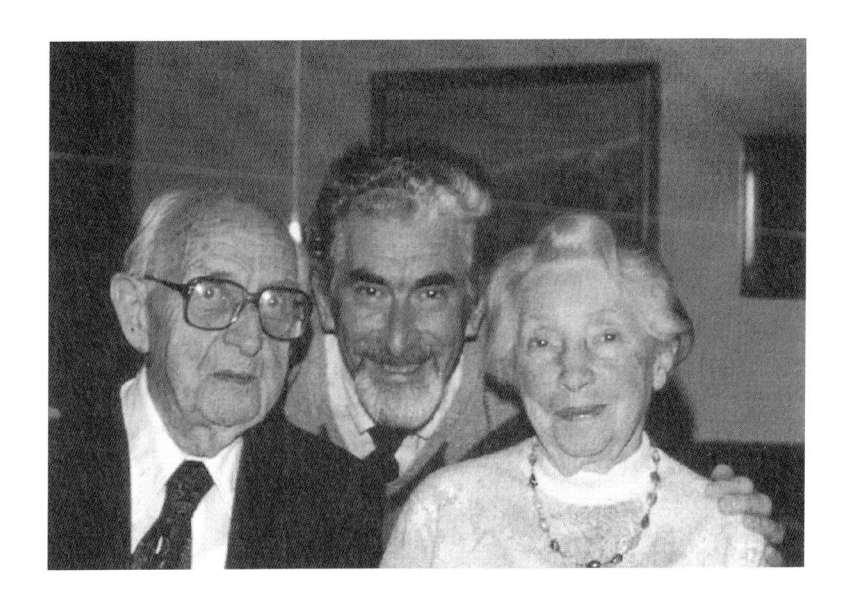

Dr. Emil Vodder † 1986

Günther Wittlinger † 1986

Estrid Vodder † 1996

This photograph was taken – 1984 at the presentation of the Rohrbach medal to Dr. Vodder by the German Association (Verband) of Physical Therapy. (VPT).

*The VPT had thus honoured a man who left us all an excellent and effective massage method.
Dr. Emil Vodder and his wife, Estrid, devoted their lives to Manual Lymph Drainage and its dissemination.
They called upon Günther Wittlinger to act as defender and advocate of Manual Lymph Drainage.*

Table of Contents

Foreword to the 2nd revised English Edition 13

Preface 15

Course of study in Manual Lymph Drainage (MLD) for health care professionals and therapists 23

Course of study in Manual Lymph Drainage (MLD) for estheticians 24

The history of Manual Lymph Drainage (MLD) 25

Part I: Theoretical Section

1	**Mode of action of Manual Lymph Drainage (MLD)**	29
1.1	Effect on the autonomic nervous system	29
1.1.1	Reflexes	30
1.2	Effect on the reflex pathways	31
1.3	Immunological effect	32
1.3.1	The immune system	32
1.3.2	Humoral immunity	33
1.3.3	Cellular immunity	34
1.4	Effect on the smooth muscles of the blood vessels and lymph angions (anatomy and function)	36
1.5	Drainage effect	40
2	**Connective tissue**	41
2.1	Structure and characteristics	41
2.2	Function	42
2.3	Connective tissue cells	44
3	**Transport systems in the body**	46
3.1	Water balance	46
3.2	Circulation	47
3.3	Lymph system	48
3.4	Lymph nodes	48
3.5	Anatomy of the lymph vessels	51
3.6	Summary of transport systems in the body	53
4	**Substance transport**	59
4.1	Molecular motion	59
4.2	Diffusion	59

Table of Contents

4.3	Substance transport in the connective tissue	60
4.4	Osmosis	60
5	**Effect of MLD on blood capillaries and connective tissue**	**61**
5.1	Structure and function of blood capillaries	61
5.2	The Starling Equilibrium	62
5.3	Effect of MLD via the blood capillaries and lymph vessels	63
6	**The significance of optimal massage pressure**	**65**
7	**Inertial Mass**	**66**
8	**Steel and rubber elasticity**	**67**
9	**The lymph vessel system**	**68**
9.1	Lymphatic watersheds	68
9.2	Anatomy and function of the initial lymph vessels	69
9.3	Protein circulation and transport	72
10	**Equilibrium and balance as a goal of massage**	**77**
10.1	Bathtub	77
10.2	Fluid equilibrium	78
10.3	Equilibrium in natural healing methods	79
11	**Oedema forms**	**80**
11.1	Lymphostatic oedema (protein-rich)	81
11.2	Dynamic oedema (low-protein)	82
11.3	Safety-valve insufficiency	84
12	**Cosmetic indications**	**85**
13	**Indications for physiotherapy**	**87**
14	**Relative contraindications (precautions)**	**88**
15	**Absolute contraindications**	**89**
16	**Treatment guidelines**	**90**
16.1	Excursus in the cosmetic field	90
16.2	Inflammations	90
16.3	Acne	92
16.4	Cellulite (panniculopathia – oedemato – fibrosclerotica)/Adiposis	92
16.5	Lipoedema	95
16.6	Toothaches	95
16.7	Consideration of outside temperature	95

16.8	Iontophoresis	96
16.9	Stress and Dr. Vodder's Manual Lymph Drainage	96
16.10	Scars	98

Part II: Practical Section

1	**Massage technique**	101
1.1	Stationary circles	101
1.2	Pump technique	101
1.3	Scoop technique	102
1.4	Rotary technique	102
1.5	Frequency of massage	102
1.6	Environmental conditions for optimal therapy	103
1.7	Basic principles	104
1.8	Sequence of manipulations	105
	I Treatment of the neck	105
	II Treatment of the face	107
	III Treatment of the arms	109
	IV Treatment of the legs	111
	V Treatment of the nape of the neck	113
	VI Treatment of the back	114
	VII Treatment of the buttocks	116
	VIII Treatment of the chest	118
	IX Treatment of the abdomen	122
	X Therapeutic movements – special techniques – oedema therapy	123
2	**Dr. Vodder on the technique of Manual Lymph Drainage**	124
2.1	Whole body treatment	125

Appendix

Lymph Drainage – A new therapeutic method serving cosmetic care ... 129

Bibliography ... 134

Foreword to the 2nd revised English Edition

Rapid scientific progress in the field of lymphology has made it necessary to update this textbook on Dr. Vodder's Manual Lymph Drainage.

We are very happy to note, at the ripe age of 86 and 87, that this book has already appeared in English, Spanish, Dutch, Italian and Swedish and is now being translated into French. This shows us that our life's work, Manual Lymph Drainage, is gradually gaining followers in many countries. Everywhere, lymph drainage has an almost magical appeal. Unfortunately, though, this demanding massage technique is also practiced by unqualified people – much to the detriment of the method. All lymph drainage teachers – both young and old – have a duty to meet at least every other year with the Dr. Vodder Schule in order to adapt theory and practice to changing requirements. We must all bear responsibility for preserving Dr. Vodder's Lymph Drainage and preventing it from becoming diluted. Our patients will benefit from our efforts. That this may always succeed is the heartfelt wish of Dr. Emil Vodder and Estrid Vodder.

Copenhagen-Bagsvaerd, July 1984   *Dr. phil. Emil Vodder*

Preface

The following preface was written by Dr. Emil Vodder, creator of the Manual Lymph Drainage method.

Although my wife and I completed the elaboration of the MLD method in France during the years 1932–1936, we were unable to write a book about it until forty years later. We have been travelling around Europe for many years now, holding lectures and courses to explain the structure and functions of the lymph system by means of drawings and manuals. Needless to say, the scientific world was not yet ready for our findings and would not accept our hypothesis and empirical evidence. The lymph system was an unknown factor in the field of physical therapy, an unexplored and dangerous *no-man's-land*. It was considered inadvisable to massage the lymphatic nodes, since it was thought that the treatment would spread bacteria and viruses. Children with swollen nodes in the neck, for example, were said to have *scrofulosis* and were operated on to remove the affected nodes. Appendicitis and spleen operations were also carried out without considering that, in so doing, the defence mechanisms of the body could be impaired – an hypothesis that later research proved to be true.

Doctors in Ancient Greece knew about the lymph system in the intestines, i.e. the chylous vessels, which resemble white chains of pearls and contain the milkywhite chylous sap. Herophilus wrote that "vessels emerging from the intestines enter a number of gland-like bodies and not the portal vein". These gland-like bodies are our lymph nodes.

In the Middle Ages anatomical research was regarded as sinful; scientific discoveries were therefore few during this period. In the Renaissance, however, a large number of important findings emerged. Many schools of anatomy were established, for example in Salerno, Bologna, Padua, Montpellier, Paris, Leyden, Copenhagen and Uppsala. In 1662, in Padua an Italian by the name of Aselli displayed the lymph vessels in a dog's intestines. He called them *chyliferi*, – shimmering milky-white veins. Six years later in London William *Harvey* published his exciting discovery, namely that the blood makes a complete circuit in the body. Two students, Jean Pecquet in Montpellier (1647) and Olaf Rudbeck in Sweden, discovered the thoracic duct in dogs. Rudbeck was a Renaissance genius who founded the still existing *Theatrum Anatomicum* in Uppsala.

Preface

In 1653 he published *Nova exercitatio anatomica* and called the newly discovered vessels *vasa serosa* and the lymph nodes *glandulae aquosae*. As a favourite of Queen Christina of Sweden, he had the honour of demonstrating his anatomical findings to the royal court.

In July 1637 a young Dane, Thomas Bartholin, was studying at the University of Leyden in Holland. His scientific research was facilitated by the existence of the *Theatrum Anatomicum* in Leyden, a library, a botanical garden and a hospital overflowing with patients. Up to that time only lunatic asylums and hospitals for plague victims had been built in Northern Europe. Bartholin studied Aselli's lymph vessels and learned how to inject gum resin and indigo into the vessels to render them visible. Over a period of ten years he visited many countries, studying languages and natural sciences. When he finally returned to Denmark he had become a renowned scientist and took over the newly built *Theatrum Anatomicum* in Copenhagen. He was the first to describe the entire lymph system. He wrote four papers in Latin, dedicated to King Frederick III, describing the lymph system as a natural process that purifies the body and regulates irritation, swelling and oedema. In *Vasa lymphatica*, 1652–1654, he describes his findings on lymph vessels and nodes in humans. No researcher had as yet used any special term for the lymph fluid. Bartholin called the vessels *vasa Lymphatica* and their content *lymph*-clear water from the Latin *limpidus*, meaning clear.

Twenty years later in Schaffhausen, Johan Conrad Peyer described the intestinal lymph aggregations, now called *Peyer's Patches*. Research was continued in many countries during the following centuries. However, Lymphology, the science of lymph and tissue fluids, was not developed until recently. The water content of the body should be studied as a whole because all organs and organic systems are intimately connected.

The ground substance is ubiquitous in the body, although it varies according to its environment, as described by Professor Hugo Grau in Dr. Zilch's instructive work, "Lymph System and Lymphatismus". This book is highly recommended to all students interested in lymph research and immunology (Munich, 1963).

Very early in our studies we were of the conviction that the human body should be regarded as a whole. We were inspired by the writings of Claude Bernard, Alexis Carrel and Cecil Drinker, who convinced us of the importance of the omnipresent lymph system in the body. Alexis Carrel, the father of modern organ transplants, confirmed this view when he received the Nobel Prize in 1912 for his research on the culti-

Preface

vation of living cells. This was an exciting period, since we foresaw what the future held for us. Carrel's classic experiment proved that the cells in a chicken's heart stayed alive if the lymph fluid was continuously renewed. Later we based our method of lymphatic regeneration of the skin on this principle. We were certain that the lymph fluid was the source of miraculous hidden forces. But despite great strides made in the field of biology, the lymphocytes retained their secret until in the middle of this century it was discovered that the nuclei of the lymphocytes contain the life-giving substance deoxyribonucleic acid (DNA), which is the prime substance of life and the vehicle of genetic traits in all organisms.

Research on the lymph system reached its peak when immunologists established that lymphocytes produce antibodies to protect the body against viruses and infections. It is of interest to note that thirty years ago one of the first lymph researchers in the United States, Professor Cecil Drinker, prophesized that the lymph system would be recognized as the most important organic system in humans and animals.

We lived eleven years of our youth in the inspiring atmosphere of France – five years on the sunny Riviera and six busy years in Paris. By studying everything that we could find about lymph and by putting what we learned into practice we were able to develop hypotheses which have long since been confirmed by researchers.

One day a client came to our physical therapy institute in Cannes for treatment of a nose and throat infection, migraine and blemished, oily skin. As usual, I closed my eyes while I palpated the hard, swollen, cervical lymph nodes. I suddenly imagined a nasal sinus covered with shimmering lymph vessels. In my mind I also saw their drainage focussed in the neck, the lymph node chains that act as a natural draining system for the skin, mucosa and meninges, i.e. for all the organs and nodes in the head and neck. As far as I know, this complex had **never** previously been interpreted as a natural separate drainage apparatus for the entire head region.

I asked myself whether obstruction in the severely swollen lymph nodes could be the underlying cause of these different ailments. Were the impurities of the skin and the catarrh of the mucous membranes the result of the malfunction of the lymph nodes? Would it be possible to unblock the drainage system by treatment with appropriate massage techniques? Had I just discovered a universal therapy to cure the lymphatic syndrome? This hypothesis has since been substantiated a

Preface

thousand times over by such treatment, which has no side-effects whatsoever. My patient was completely cured of all his ailments after ten facial massages using gentle rotary pumping movements over the lymph node chains. Nor did the ailments recur. Did the lymph have undreamt-of healing powers? No doubt!

In 1933 we moved to Paris where we continued our research, especially with regard to the anatomical and physiological aspects of the lymph vessel system. Professor Rouvière had just published his book "L'Anatomie des Lymphatiques de l'Homme" ("Anatomy of the Lymphatic Vessels in Man"). Alexis Carrel had written an invaluable book called "Der Mensch – das unbekannte Wesen" ("Man – the Unknown"), and most important was the huge atlas by the anatomist Phil. Sappey which contained a collection of very beautiful copperplate engravings, that we used a great deal during our courses in Manual Lymph Drainage. (Phil. Sappey: "Description et Iconographie des Vaisseaux Lymphatiques considérés chez l'Homme et les Vertebres", Paris 1885 – "Description and Iconography of the Lymph Vessels in Man and the Vertebrates".)

In 1936 we succeeded in compiling a simple systematic list of massage movements, using our intuition and extensive practical experience. An entirely new set of massage techniques was necessary. There had to be circular pumping and draining movements with a pressure of less than 30 mm Hg (now called Torrs) so as to **prevent** blood congestion. We employed gentle stationary circles on the lymph nodes, an area that no one had previously dared to massage, palpating with the tips or the entire length of the fingers. Massaging was always in the direction of the clavicular fossa, the terminus of all lymph pathways in the body. The method was conceived not only for facial treatment, i.e. for cosmetic and preventive measures, but also to cure illnesses. Our therapeutic treatment often produced surprising and rapid results. Positive effects were always obtained if correct, slow and rhythmic movements were employed, whether we were treating the patient for skin rejuvenation, hematomas caused by accidents, eczema, varicose veins or ulcerous legs. This was of course the fundamental principle: we were stimulating the lymph flow.

It was now time to present our findings to the public. An important exhibition took place in Paris in the spring of 1936 with a theme which particularly attracted me: Santé et Beauté ("Health and Beauty"). It was a great success, and the newspapers reported on "lymph drainage – a revolutionary skin treatment". I had written an article in French

Preface

which appeared in the Parisian journal "Santé pour Tous" ("Health for Everyone") for which I was coeditor. It was later translated into Danish and Swedish.

After spending eleven instructive years in France, we were forced to return to our home town of Copenhagen at the outbreak of the Second World War. We began again and founded a new MLD institute which we have now been running for 25 years. As we had already called the new field *lymphology*, we called the students that we trained *lymph therapists*.

But it was not until the fifties that other countries showed any interest in our work. Then we were invited to give lectures and courses in various countries, which we have now been doing for the last 20 years. We have personally trained thousands of students from Europe. We also employ assistants and a full-time staff who continue to teach our original method and life's work – "Dr. Vodder's Manual Lymph Drainage".

What progress has science made in the last decade? Modern developments such as the electron microscope, tracer methods, computers and macromolecular chemistry have also provided new insight into aspects of the lymph system for which no logical explanation had been offered till then. For example, researchers discovered the vital substance DNA in the lymphocyte nucleus, which forms the very basis of life and is the vehicle of genetic traits in all cells.

It contains the blueprints for all the tissues of our body, as already programmed in the fetus. A healthy lymph system promotes healthy body tissues and body functions. The lymph system is not only the source of good health, it also guards against infection.

Research on the lymph system, formerly known as the *neglected child of medicine*, reached its summit recently with elucidation of the immune system. Renowned lymphologists and immunologists have proved that the lymphocytes are responsible for the production of antibodies to combat viruses and infections ranging from influenza to cancer.

At the very beginning of our research my wife and I interpreted the body as a whole and thus regarded the lymph system as a source of life. The lymph system that originally developed from the primordial soup is universal and combines the macrocosmos and microcosmos within us.

Preface

It represents the omnipresent living environment of the body because all nutrients and vital substances must flow throughout the lymph interspaces by way of a *transit stretch* to the cells.

The term lymph has taken on a broad meaning in modern lymph therapy. As far as our technique is concerned it covers not only the interstitial lymph that carries the nutrient fluid to the cells but also indirectly the fluid circulating in the protoplasm of trillions of cells. It should be noted that some lymphologists insist that the connective tissue fluid is not the same as the lymph fluid. On the other hand, it is said that the lymph fluid develops in the connective tissue.

One thing, however, is certain: the lymph system not only serves to clean tissues through the drainage, but is also a protection and defense mechanism and carries out vital functions.

Just as the red blood corpuscles act as vehicles to transport oxygen and carbon dioxide, the lymph fluid carries the lymph-obligatory load (i.e. a mixture of vital substances and toxins) back to the blood stream. The lymph contains nearly all plasma-protein constituents necessary to the cells as building substances and nutrients as well as vitamins, hormones, and destroyed cells (waste products) e.g. as a result of hematomas or other injuries. Since none of these large molecules can pass through the venous walls, their transport by the lymph system is essential to life.

For this reason it is clear that the lymphocytes carry building substances to the cell tissues and that effective use of Manual Lymph Drainage can greatly accelerate the process of building new cells. Millions of lymphocytes are continuously being produced in the lymph tissues (in the palatine and pharyngeal tonsils, the spleen, the lymph nodules and *Peyer's patches*.) Recent research findings show that an average of 35 billion lymphocytes enter the blood every day through the terminal ducts that empty into large veins in the lower part of the neck. This number can increase up to as much as 562 billion during periods of stress.

Professor Collard of Brussels convincingly demonstrated the forward movement of lymph during Manual Lymph Drainage treatment. He illustrated this by means of a colour film using a contrast medium. Classical massage techniques, on the other hand, had no drainage effect whatsoever. Professor Kuhnke's investigations lead him to the same conclusions. He demonstrated that a pressure of 30 mm Hg was correct and also necessary to remove proteinacious tissue swelling (oedema). Research carried out by Casley-Smith in Australia showed that normal massage techniques are much too forceful to allow drainage in the interstitium and may hinder removal (lymph obstruction).

The lymph system is even more fascinating as a defence mechanism in the immune system and represents the most promising research field for young investigators today.

Many years ago, Professor Olliviéro, a renowned biologist in Paris, made the following humorous comparison: "Man", he said, "is an amphibian. Even the most beautiful feminine body is no more than an aquarium with 50 litres of lukewarm seawater in which trillions of cells live and fight for survival."

The unicellular organisms, which originated from the sea, have accumulated all essential chemical genetic substances on the endless road of evolution. In this aqueous environment the amoebas, or rather the lymphocytes, had to learn as unicellular organisms to protect the *private sphere*. They formed an outer covering or a membrane, so as not to be diluted or destroyed. The chemistry of life was thus protected in this fashion by the cellular membrane. Evolution, as we know it, could then begin. The existence of cells in the primordial ocean was naturally accompanied by the need for food. The cells that knew best how to exploit the energy resources flourished and gained supremacy over the less efficient cells. The best and purest source of nutrients was found in the cells themselves – harmful substances and toxins came from the exterior. Gradually some cells joined together – strength in numbers – and the inseparable cells survived.

The chemical processes that take place in the body were the best and most ingenious that mother nature could have developed. These concern the substances that regulate metabolism, i.e. sugar and fat that provide energy, amino acids that form proteins and phospholipids that make up cellular membranes.

Man has evolved unremittingly and has emerged the victor of a three-billion-year-long fight for survival.

However, the original struggle that began in the primordial ocean when the first cell turned against its own kind has never ceased despite culture, mercy and altruism.

Today we are living as always on a seabed of bacteria and viruses. The most vicious warriors measure only seven microns in diameter and yet are our deadliest foes. These tiny enemies carry out silent lightning

Preface

attacks. Viruses and bacteria that enter a cut finger or the mucous membrane can reach the brain cells seconds later. For this very reason our immune system maintains a huge arsenal of white blood corpuscles. A person weighing 70 kilograms has an average of 26 billion granulocytes and macrophages (phagocytes) from the bone marrow at the ready. In addition there are other groups of chemical *guards* and microbiological *killer cells*. Professor Gowans of Oxford stated in a lecture: "There is no doubt that our ability to survive in an environment full of hostile microorganisms depends on the strength of our huge army of lymphocytes."

As a preface to this first textbook I have written a retrospective report on the development of Manual Lymph Drainage (MLD) and have also provided an outline of scientific efforts aimed at disclosing the all-important secrets of the lymph system. We express our deep gratitude to Mr. and Mrs. Wittlinger, the directors of the Dr. Vodder School in Walchsee, Tirol, for meeting a long-felt need with this textbook.

Copenhagen-Bagsvaerd, January 1978   *Dr. phil. Emil Vodder*

Course of study in Manual Lymph Drainage (MLD) for health care professionals and therapists

The program for therapists lasts for four weeks (180 units) and is divided into a basic part (also known as Basic & Therapy I courses) and a therapy part (also known as Therapy II and III). After successful completion, the therapist is able to treat those disorders indicated for MLD (including oedema therapy). The diploma awarded to the students upon passing the examination of the Dr. Vodder School, Walchsee, is internationally recognized.

Graduates of the course pledge themselves to continued education in MLD, as new findings on the effect of MLD and continuous practical reviews of the manual techniques make this essential.

Weekend courses or so called Review courses are also held for therapists with the aim of promoting continued training. Good technique is decisive for therapeutic success. The Dr. Vodder School, Walchsee, teaches the original method.

Course of study in Manual Lymph Drainage (MLD) for estheticians

Training in Manual Lymph Drainage comprises basic, advanced and review courses.

- There is a **basic neck & face course**.
    Part 1: treatment of the neck
    Part 2: treatment of the face
  Each part is accompanied by theory, making a total of 20 hours.

- The **advanced neck & face course** refines the techniques of the basic neck and face class and prepares the student for the theory and practical exam, given at the end of the course. Students are taught esthetic applications of MLD for the neck and face. This course is also 20 hours.

- The **basic body course** is divided into four parts:
    Part 1: treatment of the neck and face.
    Part 2: treatment of the arms and legs.
    Part 3: treatment of the nape of the neck, back and loin.
    Part 4: treatment of the breast and abdomen.

  Each part is accompanied by a theoretical hour, making a total of 40 hours of instruction for the basic course.

- The **advanced body course** refines the techniques learned in the basic course and prepares the student in both theoretical and practical aspects for the final examination given at the end of the advanced course. In addition, special practical applications in cosmetics are covered. Upon passing the examination, which is divided into a theoretical and practical part, the student receives an internationally recognised diploma that entitles him or her to practice MLD independently in the fields of health care and cosmetics. The advanced course consists of 40 hours of instruction.

- **Review courses**, lasting two or more days are offered for improving technique, exchanging practical experience, and extending theoretical knowledge.

The history of Manual Lymph Drainage (MLD)

In 1932 Dr. Vodder and his wife were working as massage therapists in Cannes on the French Riviera. The majority of their patients were English who were there to recover from chronic colds, caused by the damp climate in Britain. The Vodders discovered that all of the patients had swollen lymph nodes in their necks. At that time the lymphatic system was taboo for massage therapists – even for physicians. The prevailing view was to take no note whatsoever of it. It was regarded as a medical Pandora's box. Vodder dared to break the taboo and treated the swollen lymph nodes intuitively and successfully. The colds vanished. Encouraged by these successes, he developed the MLD method as we teach and apply it today.

His method was first made known to the public in 1935 and his first publication appeared in 1936 in Paris [1]. From this time on – for 40 years – he remained active as a massage therapist, held lectures, gave demonstration treatments with his wife and taught courses. Also, the term "Manual Lymph Drainage" was coined by the Vodders. This gives them the claim as the originators.

Attracted by these pioneering activities, a growing number of massage therapists, estheticians and physicians became interested in MLD. This led in 1967 to the founding of the "Society for Dr. Vodder's Manual Lymph Drainage", whose aim was to scientifically substantiate the effect of MLD and to set up optimal courses of study for the various professional groups.

In the next chapter, the scientific basis of MLD will be presented with special attention given to the question: Can the therapist use MLD? (For the therapist the book contains all the subject matter of the basic course.)

The Society for Dr. Vodder's MLD, founded in 1967, was integrated in 1976 into the German Society of Lymphology as the section Therapeutic Lymph Drainage and Cosmetic Dermatological Lymph Drainage. The heritage was assumed by the Society for Dr. Vodder's Lymph Drainage in Walchsee, which was established in 1972. The Dr. Vodder School founded at the same place teaches the unaltered original method. The goal of this school is to incorporate MLD into the training, and to supervise the teachers in order to ensure that people benefit

The history of Manual Lymph Drainage (MLD)

from the method. The objectives of the school are in full accordance with the wishes of Dr. Vodder and his instructions to the authors.

The following chapters do not claim to be complete. They are intended as an aid to the esthetician and therapist in understanding the complex scientific basis of how MLD works. For this reason we have chosen a somewhat simplified approach.

Part I
Theoretical Section

1 Mode of action of Manual Lymph Drainage (MLD)

1.1 Effect on the autonomic nervous system

We know that MLD acts on the body in various ways. MLD acts on the **autonomic nervous system**. This consists of the sympathetic nervous system, the day nerve, which makes us active and allows us to work, and the parasympathetic system, the night nerve, which permits us to rest, sleep, and renew our strength for the next day.

These two nerves extend to all parts of the body; that is to say, vessels, muscles, organs, and – especially interesting to the esthetician – the skin, and exert an equalizing effect that is vital to the very existence of the organism [9a]. We find branches (axons) of the autonomic nervous system in the soft connective tissue ground substance.

In a healthy person the autonomic nervous system is balanced. Daily stress, the environment, striving for success are factors contributing to the fact that many of us no longer possess balanced autonomic systems. As a result, the sympathetic nervous system predominates.

MLD, on the other hand, has a calming effect on the sympathetic nervous system. This means that after proper application of MLD the patient becomes calmer, more relaxed some even fall asleep during treatment. This effect is desirable, for many women come to the esthetician just to enjoy an hour of relaxation. They like to be looked after and attended to. Their pleasure is increased by the effect of MLD. There are a number of patients whose disease stems from the fact that they are in a state of disharmony in which the sympathetic system dominates. Hutzschenreuter [48] writes that MLD can have a *sympathicolytic* effect (i.e. calming on the sympathetic system.).

MLD is at least one of the possible types of therapies that can successfully be used in these cases.

It is therefore essential that the manual techniques be carried out in a slow, monotonous rhythm. If performed too quickly, they will have just the opposite effect; they will stimulate the patient and make her/him nervous. The parasympathetic system has a trophotropic effect; that is, it promotes growth and recovery and restores strength. These are pro-

1 Mode of action of Manual Lymph Drainage (MLD)

cesses that are characteristic of sleep and cannot be influenced by conscious will. The causes of muscular hypertension [2] are often of a subconscious nature. Our conscious mind is subordinate to the motor and sensory functions of the body. If the hypertension of many of our clients were not caused by the subconscious, they could consciously control or influence the disorder themselves. This, however is not the case. In using MLD, we are able to influence muscular hypertension through the autonomic nervous system.

Whereas the conscious mind in man is centered in the cerebrum, the sources of unconscious nonphysical stimuli are assumed to be seated in the autonomic centres of the rest of the brain and the spinal column. Reflexes that can be triggered by physical manipulation act upon autonomic centres.

One of the great physician-massage therapists, Dr. H. Marnitz [26], wrote: Dr. Vodder's Lymph Drainage is based on an ingeniously devised, simple and convincing technique that brings about an acceleration of lymph flow. At the same time, however, a soothing effect on the sensitive nerve endings of the skin is achieved and a certain reflex detonization of the skin.

1.1.1 Reflexes

A reflex [3] is a response to a stimulus. Nerve cells called receptors are organs designed to receive various kinds of stimulus. For example, there are receptors that respond to light, chemical substances, heat, and mechanical influences. The receptor converts the stimulus it is designed to receive into an electrical signal and transmits it to a nerve cell. The nerve cell then conveys the signal via axons to the reflex centres. From this switching point, the signals are relayed to the respective target organs. For example, when you prick your finger with a needle, the target organs are those muscles that pull your finger away. Many reflexes are accompanied by feelings. The reflexes that are of interest to us are the fight or flight reflexes as well as those that induce pleasure. Hard, rough massaging may set off recoil and defence reactions or even flight reflexes. The resulting pain is usually associated with increased muscle tension. Feelings of aversion (e.g. anger, fear) accompany these reflexes.

When MLD is properly employed, however, pleasure reflexes are elicited. These are accompanied by pleasant sensations (e.g. feelings of affection, well being). They lower the basic activity of the muscles and thus exert a relaxing effect.

1.2 Effect on the reflex pathways [3]

The nerves known as nociceptive fibres transmit pain-causing stimuli from the periphery in the form of action potentials. The word nociceptive comes from the Latin nocere (to hurt). If you put a rubber band around your wrist, then pull it and let it snap back, you will feel pain. After some time a red welt appears that swells. We have here all the symptoms of inflammation: swelling, reddening, pain, and heat. This is the local response to a pain stimulus, which is received by a nociceptor (pain receptor) and is transmitted in the form of action potential via nociceptive fibres, the spinal column, and the brain stem to the cerebrum. The pain stimulus results from the destruction of cells in the affected area. The breakdown products of the destroyed cells, such as histamine, serotonin, and prostaglandins, act on the nociceptive fibres. It is this that then produces in us the sensation we call pain.

A nociceptive stimulus is received by the appropriate receptor, a nociceptor, and transmitted by way of nerves to the point of transition to the next ganglion cell. This transition point is called a synapse. In this case the synapse transmits a stimulation. It is excitatory and is able to convey the excitation to the higher areas of the central nervous system.

The nociceptor continues to send action potentials to the central nervous system as long as it is excited; that is, as long as the cause of the pain persists.

Besides nociceptors, there are also touch receptors. These transmit stimuli produced by touch, such as those that are elicited by MLD or stroking. They too transmit these touch sensations by means of action potentials via nerves to the vertebral column. There they encounter ganglion cells, whose synapses also have an excitatory function. The stimulus is relayed via axons of the ganglion cell to higher areas of the central nervous system, where the agreeable sensation of touch is elicited. The axon possesses a collateral; that is, a connection that leads to another ganglion cell. This ganglion cell is known as an inhibitory cell. Upon being stimulated, it transmits the action potential to the ganglion cell that is excited by the nociceptor. Together, these two ganglion cells form an inhibitory synapse, which means that any pain signals coming

1 Mode of action of Manual Lymph Drainage (MLD)

from the nociceptors are inhibited, blocked, or even cancelled, whenever the inhibitory cell is simultaneously excited. There is, however, one reservation: the touch receptor responds only to changes in the stimulus.

Thus, it is continuously excited by MLD, since the constantly changing pressure applied during MLD brings along a continuous variation in the stimulation. In this way the touch receptors – and thus the inhibitory cells – are continuously excited.

In simple terms, this means that precise execution of MLD, which is characterised by light, continually changing pressure, activates inhibitory cells whose function is to decrease or even eliminate sensations of pain.

At this point, we should like to mention that MLD's drainage effect can likewise alleviate pain – as for instance in the cases of hematomas or distortions (sprains), with consequent local swelling. The affected region is painful, due partly to the swelling and partly to substances in the connective tissue which stimulate the nociceptors. Both of these are positively affected by MLD.

1.3 Immunological effect

1.3.1 The immune system

With MLD we treat all lymph nodes that are accessible to our hands. Thus, we treat some of the most important organs of the body's immune system. Nowadays we must familiarise ourselves with various terms of immunology, although we might not be able to prove that MLD influences the body's immunity. "What does the immune system protect?" [22] The immune system distinguishes between self and nonself. In the body the feature self is carried to a large extent by proteins, but also polysaccharides and lipids. In the larger molecules of multicellular animals certain chemical groups possess a spatial arrangement that is characteristic of the species. This species-specific spatial pattern within the molecule is the genetically coded self feature. It is by virtue of this special molecular arrangement that every living species claims its uniqueness. It is the function of the immune system to protect this uniqueness.

The immune system is directed not only against infectious pathogens, i.e. their virulence, but also against substances that are foreign to the species, especially proteins. Only pathogens (bacteria and viruses) that possess virulence, antigenity, or both will trigger the defence mechanisms of the immune system.

In addition, the immune system is responsible for getting rid of body tissue that no longer has a function, as this represents a disturbing influence in the protein individuality of the organism.

The immune system constitutes a vital protective system of the body. **Immunity** is understood to be the protection we have against a second attack of an infectious disease.

Thus, a person contracts measles only once in life because the body is immune after the disease has abated. Immunity against measles, however, does not protect us against other infectious diseases. This property of immunity is known as specificity.

Two mechanisms are responsible for immunity. First, proteins (globulins) are the vehicles of the defence function. These are called antibodies; they are the mediators of **humoral immunity**. Second, there are cells (lymphocytes, plasma cells, phagocytes, macrophages) that can render detrimental substances harmless. We call this **cellular immunity**.

1.3.2 Humoral immunity

There are numerous interactions between the two systems (humoral and cellular) [4]. There are numerous antigenic substances, including various pathogens, that are able to provoke an immune reaction. Furthermore, antigens have the ability to react specifically with an antibody or a sensitized lymphocyte. Antibodies are present in all body fluids: in the blood, the lymph, and in loose connective tissue [5]. These antibodies, which are formed primarily in the lymph nodes, have learned to react against very specific invaders. Antibodies are globulin molecules, which can be separated into five different fractions by means of a special chemical process called *immunoelectrophoresis*. Immunoglobulin A (IgA) and immunoglobulin G (IgG) have substantial protective properties against viruses, bacteria, and mutant cells of the body itself. Immunoglobulin M (IgM) (for macro) reacts especially quickly. It represents the *shock troop* of our defence system. Then comes immunoglobulin G (IgG) followed by IgA whose protective

1 Mode of action of Manual Lymph Drainage (MLD)

effect is less rapid but more sustained. IgE is especially important in the case of allergies. IgA occurs above all in mucous membranes and has the function of fending off the attackers at the portal of entry – before they can enter the body fluid or the lymph system. IgA [6], produced by plasma cells, is provided with a secretory portion of epithelial cells and mixed with the secretion of the mucosa. It is found in saliva, tears, milk, and colostrum and in the wastes of the gastrointestinal, urogenital, and respiratory tracts. These immunoglobulins are not produced and presented to the same degree in all people. One thing is certain: lymphostasis (blockage of the lymph) can prevent the immunoglobulins from reaching the sites where they are needed. Thus, in the protein molecules there are defence functions [5] that we all possess, and in the lymph vessels and lymph nodes there is a special defence reaction that results from the synthesis of specifically acting antibody globulins. Although they are all immunoglobulins, each is designed to put one particular opponent out of action.

Proteins are produced by the liver [7], which receives the building blocks of proteins, namely amino acids and peptides, from the intestinal wall via the bloodstream. Albumins are released by the liver directly into the bloodstream, but globulins are stored in certain cellular systems (plasma cells, macrophages, lymphocytes, thymus gland, reticular cells of the spleen, and in connective tissue). From there they can be dispatched – independently of the variable protein supply in the diet – into the bloodstream to meet the immunological needs of the body.

To a lesser extent, the kidneys, spleen and lymph system are also involved in the synthesis of proteins from amino acids received in the diet. It is therefore essential that protein be supplied at meals to satisfy the body's needs. At the same time, however, a constant high-protein diet should be discouraged on the grounds that if continued over extended periods, it may lead to hypoporopathy (lowered permeability of capillary membranes due to thickening).

1.3.3 Cellular immunity

The cellular defence of the body is mediated by lymphocytes [4], plasma cells, macrophages, and phagocytes. Lymphocytes are especially numerous in the lymph nodes, spleen, Peyer's patches and tonsils. Within the lymph nodes a distinction is made between the outer, cortical and the inner, medullary zones. In the cortical zone we find predominantly lymphocytes arranged in spherical follicles, which may also populate the paracortical zones situated between the follicles near the venules. The medullus consists primarily of macrophages and plasma cells aligned in filaments around the lymph sinus.

Two types of lymphocytes are known: T lymphocytes and B lymphocytes [8]. These cells do not originate in the spleen or in the lymph nodes. They migrate into these organs during an early phase of development, but are found originally in the red bone marrow. T lymphocytes receive their characteristic features from thymosin of the thymus gland, through which they pass on their way from the bone marrow to the lymphoid complex. B lymphocytes are given their characteristic traits by the Peyer's patches.

T and B lymphocytes are morphologically indistinguishable [4]. Both appear as small and large lymphocytes. The most important distinction is the presence of immunoglobulins on the surface of B cells, which are not detectable on T cells. On the surface of a B lymphocyte are identical immunoglobins of one and the same type, all having the same specificity for one particular antigen. Whenever a cell of this type encounters its corresponding antigen, an antigen-antibody reaction takes place on its surface. The lymphocyte then differentiates and upon completing a series of divisions becomes either a plasma cell or a small lymphocyte again. The plasma cell then produces and secretes antibodies.

Upon coming into contact once again with its antigen, the lymphocyte recognizes it with the help of its surface receptors and changes into a blast. This is the vehicle of the immunological memory and is known as the memory cell.

T lymphocytes can kill directly; they are responsible for cellular defence. They usually assist the B cells in recognizing antigens.

The maturation stages of lymphocytes can be divided into three functional categories of the lymph system:

1. Stem cells are formed in the bone marrow.

2. Cells mature and are transformed into T and B lymphocytes.

3. In the lymphatic organs – spleen, lymph nodes, Peyer's patches, tonsils – B and T lymphocytes are found in various ratios. These are immunologically competent against all antigens.

1 Mode of action of Manual Lymph Drainage (MLD)

Still another cell is involved in the immunological response: the macrophage. Unlike lymphocytes it is unspecific in its action. The immunological benefit of MLD resides in the fact that pathogenic substances present in the body fluids are transported rapidly by manual manipulation to the lymph nodes, where they are deactivated. Generally speaking [6], successful defence against infection by microorganisms depends on the degree of **resistance** and the presence of immunity. Resistance is understood to be the entire defence complex that the body can mobilise against the antigens of a pathogen before the immunological response is initiated. Resistance is not antigen-specific. It is determined by genetic and environmental factors (such as nutrition, exhaustion, disease). There is no doubt that resistance is strengthened by regular MLD.

We also know through observation that we influence immunological events and that the treatment of mucous membranes with MLD yields good results. This is because we maintain or even improve the habitat of IgA antibodies.

1.4 Effect on the smooth muscles of the blood vessels and lymph angions (anatomy and function)

MLD can have a tonic effect on the smooth muscles of the blood vessel [9]. One theory is that the tissue pressure on the small arteries is lowered due to the drainage effect of MLD in the connective tissue. These small vessels only have sparsely developed musculature and are thus quite sensitive to tissue pressure. If this pressure should drop, the amplitude of the capillary pulsation increases and is followed by an increase in the speed of capillary blood flow. This increase in the rate of flow is accompanied by increased metabolic changes and resorption around the capillary. The tissue is then emptied.

The lymph vessels are constructed differently from the blood vessels (draw and compare the two). It was Aselli who in 1622 first observed contractions of the lymph vessels in dogs. It was not until 300 years later, in 1956 that spontaneous rhythmical contractions of the lymph vessels in man were described by Kinmonth and Taylor.

If we liken the blood vessels to pipes that are made up of three layers (intima, media, and adventia), the lymph vessels can be said to re-

Effect on the smooth muscles of the blood vessels 1.4

semble a small heart in construction. Accordingly, the lymph vessels are built up of individual valved segments, called lymph angions by Mislin, which are to be interpreted as anatomical and functional units. Each of these lymphatic segments has a on-way valve that determines the direction of lymph flow and prevents backflow. The spiral and ring-shaped smooth muscles of the segments contract in response to various stimuli and press the contents of the lymph vessels, the lymph, in the direction in which the valves open.

The innervation of the lymph vessels has been investigated by many researchers. It has been concluded that stimulation of various nerves leads to contraction of the lymph vessels, either actively or reactively. Mechanoreceptors have also been found in the lymph vessel wall. It may therefore be stated that the lymph volume in the peripheral lymph vessels determines the pulsation rate and thus the transport rate of the lymph. Other factors are stimuli produced by:

- Movements of the skeletal muscles.
- Pulsation of the arteries.
- The pressure difference in the thorax created by breathing.
- Peristaltic movements of the intestine.
- Manual Lymph Drainage.

These stimuli are known as auxiliary pumps, which work on vessel walls from the outside.

Apart from this the lymph angion also has a possibility of *self* contraction. It contracts between 3 and 7 times per minute (autonomous or autochthonous).

The pulsation rate of the lymph vessels fluctuates between 1 and 30 pulses per minute, whereby a relation between intravascular pressure and contraction rate has been established. It is important to note here that contractility of the vessel walls is also dependent on the tonus of the wall.

The chief influence on pulsation, however, comes from stretching. As described earlier this can come from inside, i.e. by filling, and/or by stretching the vessel from outside. Mislin has proved experimentally that an increased contraction is produced by stretching the lymph angion lengthwise and transversely. Moving the skin during Vodder's special Lymph Drainage technique creates this lengthwise and diagonal stretching of the lymph vessels and thus leads to an increased contraction.

1 Mode of action of Manual Lymph Drainage (MLD)

An increase of the lymphangio-motoricity (vessel pulsation) will however always result in an acceleration of lymph flow. It is the task of the lymph vessels to maintain the flow of lymph. According to Hutzschenreuter, lymph transport is understood as the forward movement of lymph in the lymph collectors via the main lymph trunks. These include the thoracic duct and the left and right intercostal trunks, etc. Peripherally, lymph transport takes place actively by means of contractions of the lymph angions; in the vicinity of the main lymph trunks, it is primarily due to pressure variations in the abdomen and thorax.

Now let us visualise that the fluids within the individual body cavities are in constant motion. This occurs as circulation within the spaces and as diffusion, osmosis, filtration or active transport across the borders of these cavities.

Since every fluid cavity constitutes a continuous system, the fluid within them is freely mobile. Factors that tend to impair free circulation are the resistance caused by friction along the adjacent cells and the internal friction associated with specific properties of the fluid, i.e. the viscosity of the fluid. The chief causes of circulation are the concentration and osmotic gradients and differences in the density of the medium which is dependent on the temperature gradients in the individual cavities. Most important are the mechanical, motor driving forces.

When body compartments are constructed and arranged in such a way that the mechanical forces can and do give rise to regular movements of fluid, we speak of a circulatory system. Typically, the fluid flows through sharply delineated channels, tubes or vessels. When vessels contract actively, as the lymph vessels do, they then play an important part in fluid transport – in this case lymph drainage.

A closer look at lymph drainage reveals that there are three types:

1. Extravascular lymph drainage involves lymph formation and extravascular circulation. Lymph is formed from: blood plasma which finds its way into the interstitial spaces by filtration or diffusion, from various proteins which enter the interstitial spaces mainly by active transport (cytopemphis), from large-molecular fat molecules from the digestive tract, from non-migratory cells (see also lymph-obligatory load). The more protein there is in the tissue, the less water can flow out of the tissue via the venous blood capillaries, because protein retains the water. By transporting protein out of the interstitial spaces, the lymph system again permits more water to flow out through the blood capillaries.

2. Extramural lymph drainage, i.e. the external mechanical influences on the lymph vessel. This is based on the fact that specific external forces, as described, stimulate the angio-motoricity.

3. Auxiliary, indirect lymph drainage, which is supported locally or regionally by manual, direct lymph drainage.

   To cite Mislin in one of his lectures: "If Manual Lymph Drainage did not yet exist, it would have to be invented as it is now performed". I think this says everything about the effectiveness of MLD.

Mislin has also described how the unique manipulations of MLD stimulate the lymphatic motor system: Physiologic vasomotor lymph drainage is based on the autonomic pulsations of the lymph angion or chain of lymph angions. MLD probably exerts a decisive influence on this system of drainage. The pulsation is comprised of repeating, sequential, rhythmic dilations and contractions of a group of lymph segments. The dilation-contraction frequency of the segments is synchronized. The resultant pulsation is a sequential peristalsis. Synergistic-functioning receptors in the vessel walls enable myogenic automation and control of vascular activity. This ensures a coordinated lymph transport. The main physiologic stimuli are pressure and temperature stimuli. Intravascular transversal, but also longitudinal, stretching stimuli increase the *pulse* rate of the lymph sections. Smooth muscle cells, such as those in the vessel wall, exhibit electrical and mechanical reactions after undergoing passive stretching. A specific stretching is required for vessel wall muscles that exhibit autonomic, i.e. pacemaking characteristics. Their stimulation is thus regulated according to prevailing conditions. The degree of stretching depends on the degree to which the vessels are filled. As MLD provides a tensile stimulation (to a certain extent inadequate), MLD thus stimulates vasomotor lymph drainage.

We achieve this with the special lymph drainage technique of Dr. Vodder. The total pumping capacity of the lymph vessels is provided by the sum of the lymphatic segments. An increase in intralymphatic pressure can also result in an increase in the lymph pulse rate. The rate of lymph flow increases with an increased lymph-obligatory load. This means that increased lymph production, or to say it differently: the capacity of transport of the lymph vessel system is increased by a higher lymph-time-volume.

1 Mode of action of Manual Lymph Drainage (MLD)

1.5 Drainage effect [29]

The term drainage certainly did not originate in biology, but rather, strictly speaking, from farming and agriculture. Here it refers to the method, first practiced in England, of converting marshy land to farmland by the removal of excess water. Throughout the Middle Ages, however, no mention is made of draining waterlogged soil. Not until the middle of the 18th century is land drainage mentioned. Relatively late in the 18th century reference is made to drainage systems, in which subsurface conduits are used to collect and dispose of water. True drain systems employ two types of conduits; field drains and collection drains. Field drains are designed to remove the water directly from the soil. Groups of field drains then discharge the water into a collection drain. The field drains are generally laid out in parallel fashion, with the system being cross-connected to some extent by lateral conduits. A further feature of drainage was the drain plan, i.e. the drainage system was laid out in accordance with the features of the area to be reclaimed. As a rule the drainage area of a drainage conduit increases substantially with the depth at which it is laid. Naturally, the actual conduit diameter depends on the volume of water to be removed. The drainage or drain plan changes, depending on the terrain and the stratification of the soil. The preflood features of the drainage area in particular determine the size of the main conduit.

The initial lymph drainage system is laid out according to the same criteria that have been tested and used in agriculture. The initial lymph vessels serve as field drains and the lymph vessels of various orders as collection drains.

Brunner designated lymph vessels of various calibre as lymph vessels of 1st, 2nd or 3rd order [32].

When we speak of drainage in connection with MLD, we are referring to the removal of fluid from soft connective tissue. Thus we transport water and substances from loose connective tissue via the lymph vessel system. These substances are referred to as the lymph-obligatory load. Some water is also removed via the blood vessel system.

Since this effect is of crucial importance to all professional groups using MLD, it will be treated in detail in a later section.

2 Connective tissue

2.1 Structure and characteristics

Connective tissue is partly comprised of bone and cartilage, the hard supporting substance, partly of taut connective tissue, including tendons and fascia, and partly of loose connective tissue rich in cells, e.g. the subcutis. When we mention connective tissue here in relation to MLD, we mean the loose connective tissue, the binding tissue that joins the cells together to form tissue groups. These tissue groups join to form organs, and finally the organs form an organism. Loose connective tissue is made up of several substances, including the ground substance, consisting of: proteins as the soluble precursors of collagen; non-collagenous proteins which form protein-polysaccharide complexes, mucopolysaccharides; hyaluronic acid; hyaluronidase; chondroitin sulphuric acid; the various cellular elements, such as fibroblasts, from which small and large reticular cells arise; small and large round cells; histiocytes; resting migratory cells; chondrocytes; lymphocytes; plasma cells; granulocytes; mast cells and fat cells. The migratory cells of the connective tissue are able to detach themselves from the tissue matrix. They then become mobile and are especially capable of phagocytosis.

Various fibres are also components of connective tissue: collagenous, elastic and reticular fibres.

Further constituents include blood capillaries and initial lymph vessels and the end fibres of the autonomic nervous system. The nerves, vessels and parenchyma cells form a triad which is capable of initiating regulation processes in the connective tissue. These regulation processes concern the functions and abilities of connective tissue. MLD, a massage form adapted to this type of tissue, helps to normalise the function and composition of connective tissue. This is achieved because with the special MLD method, fluid and solutes in the connective tissue can be displaced extravasally in any desired direction.

The connective tissue is composed of up to 70% water and is moveable and varies in its viscosity. To cite an example from chemistry, one could say it has thixotrophic properties. The following experiment illustrates an example of thixotrophic behaviour:

Bentonite and water mixed in the proper proportions yield a mass which also has thixotrophic properties. If this mass is shaken in a bottle it will become fluid, but if allowed to stand for a while after shaking, it

2 Connective tissue

will become gelatinous. Thixotrophy is the mechanical transformation of a substance from a gel to a sol and back. We should add here that in every cubic centimetre of connective tissue we also have other structures present.

If we apply appropriate distortion forces to the connective tissue in terms of pressure and skin movement (e.g. light vibrations or MLD), then we can free the connective tissue of substances affecting it or that are causing disease. MLD has the following effects on the connective tissue: the connective tissue is purified with small molecular substances and water being resorbed into the blood stream. By stimulating the lymphangio-motoricity, the large molecular substances (we include here the waste metabolites and the whole lymph-obligatory load and toxins) are removed from the connective tissue.

The *lymph-obligatory* load includes all substances in the connective tissue which because of their molecular size can only be transported through the lymph system. We describe here protein, cell, water and fat loads and include glass, mineral or coal dust as well as bacteria.

2.2 Function

Connective tissue is an organ and as such has many functions and capabilities. It is the vehicle of the unconscious and undifferentiated bodily functions. It regulates energy processes and primarily controls the physiochemical and bioelectrical situation. It thus regulates such vital functions as temperature, water, mineral and energy balance, including glycolysis and respiration. It forms the basis of the system of general and unspecific defence regulation and along with its fibres represents a mechanical barrier for bacteria.

Wendt [24] has shown that connective tissue also serves as the physiologic reservoir of the human body for all essential nutrients. Protein, carbohydrates and water are stored in the connective tissue as well as fat cells which contain fat not yet transformed into energy. Excess dietary protein is stored in collagen and the amino group of the mucopolysaccharide molecule. Water is stored within the structure of this molecule in the connective tissue. Carbohydrates are stored in two different water-insoluble polysaccharide molecules; partly in glycogen, a pure polysaccharide that is mainly found in the liver and muscle cells, and partly in the amino sugars called mucopolysaccharides, which are found in connective tissue and the basement membrane. The mucopolysaccharides in the connective tissue represent the main carbohydrate reservoir of the body. The mucopolysaccharides in connective tissue vary according to the amount and type of food ingested; its sugar content is in any case considerably larger than that of the glycogen reservoir in the liver and muscles, which only lasts from one meal to the next. Glycogen synthesis is under the influence of insulin; mucopolysaccharide synthesis is not.

Water occurs in two different forms in the body: 1. as active, hydrodynamic, available water and 2. as inactive, stored water. The first form serves as a means of transport in the circulatory and lymph system as well as in connective tissue. It functions as a reactive partner and as a solvent in metabolic processes of cells and tissues. The stored water, on the other hand is bound by the fibrils of the mucopolysaccharide molecules and is inactivated. It determines the volume of the molecule, which is not a compact but rather a diffused, externally open molecule that extends over a large volume, its so-called domain.

The vitamin and mineral content of the stored nutrients also fulfills a storage function. The calcium reservoir is bone, which is also a type of connective tissue. The calcium is stored in the form of calcium phosphate and calcium carbonate molecules. Evolution has placed this central reservoir for all nutrients in the most imaginably convenient spot in the body – the connective tissue. In this way the connective tissue fulfills two functions. First, it is an hydroculture in which all cells of the body are suspended and nourished. Second, it is the ubiquitous reservoir for all the nutrients of the entire organism. In this way, every body cell can withdraw any nutrient from the tissue fluid in which it is bathed. If a nutrient deficiency occurs, every cell can at any time draw nutrients out of the omnipresent reservoir without any delay due to long transport routes.

Some people are of the opinion that connective tissue be viewed solely as a passive transit stretch for the transport of substances from the capillary to the cell and back. Pischinger [9a] however, calls the connective tissue an organ. This leads to the term cell-milieu system, which means that the life quality of the cells is dependent upon their environment. We consider the latter view logical. Evidence for this view is the presence of nerve fibres in the soft connective tissue, in which the termination of the autonomic nerves. The axons of these nerves are able to release transmitter substances directly into the connective tissue, thereby exerting a regulatory effect.

2 Connective tissue

A further characteristic of connective tissue is its ability to regenerate, for example, the formation of scars (fibroblasts).

Connective tissue has yet another important function as a defence system against life-threatening invasions from foreign cells, e.g. bacteria. The connective tissue fibres represent a protective barrier that detains invading cells until the defence cells can do their work. Fatty tissue is a type of connective tissue, serving both as a reservoir and as padding.

Extracellular tissue, pericapillary tissue, transit stretch, interstitium and basic regulatory tissue are various names for one and the same thing: the connective tissue. The different names for this tissue reflect its multiple functions. From this it follows that a good healthy connective tissue is essential for health and beauty. An accumulation of metabolic waste products impairs the function of connective tissue. In milder cases this leads to cosmetic blemishes, in serious cases to health disturbances. The same is true if disturbances occur in the water balance of connective tissue or if its composition deviates from the norm. As a scientist has said just recently: "One may assume that micro-oedemas in connective tissue are the cause of many diseases."

2.3 Connective tissue cells

Connective tissue contains cells that not only produce collagen and elastic fibres but also a ubiquitous half-gel, half-fluid, binding mass which is a part of the ground substance. It is through this ground substance that transport takes place: the transport of nutrients from the blood capillaries to the cell and the transport of waste products from the cell to the capillaries. The connective tissue cell has all of the enzymes necessary for the synthesis of collagen [10], elastin and polysaccharide proteins. It can quickly produce several times its own weight in extracellular substance. The connective tissue cells can only be supplied with building blocks by a suitable diet consisting of nutrient-rich foods plus oxygen. Parenchyma cells are surrounded by ground substance which is involved in nourishing these cells. The condition of the ground substance will affect the rate of diffusion through it. In a sense, it is the environment for the cells.

This environment can be clean and healthy or polluted with metabolic wastes and unhealthy. It is easy to imagine that the cells fare better in a healthy milieu. MLD cleans and purifies the tissue by draining it of pollutants [30].

Hyaluronic acid is a constituent of the ground substance. Hyaluronidase is the enzyme that breaks down hyaluronic acid. These two substances occur in the body in equal amounts. This equilibrium ensures that synthesis and breakdown balance each other. The addition of hyaluronidase would upset this equilibrium. Hyaluronic acid also serves as cement for the filaments of the initial lymph vessels [11]. The use of hyaluronidase in the form of creams, salves, injections, tablets or infiltrative liquids dissolves this cement on the filaments and causes insufficiency of the initial lymph vessels. In beauty care, the use of substances containing hyaluronidase should therefore be strongly discouraged.

3 Transport systems in the body

3.1 Water balance

The body consists of one-third solid substances and two-thirds of a liquid similar to seawater, evidence that we originally evolved from marine life.

When we take a closer look at the liquid, we find it consists of 5% blood, 15% connective tissue fluid and 40–45% intracellular fluid. The fluids are vital to us because substances can only be transported in a liquid milieu. Health is often dependent on the circulation of substances (metabolism), and is therefore a matter of adequate transport. The drawing shows the blood separated from the intracellular fluid by connective tissue. This is intentionally so represented, since all

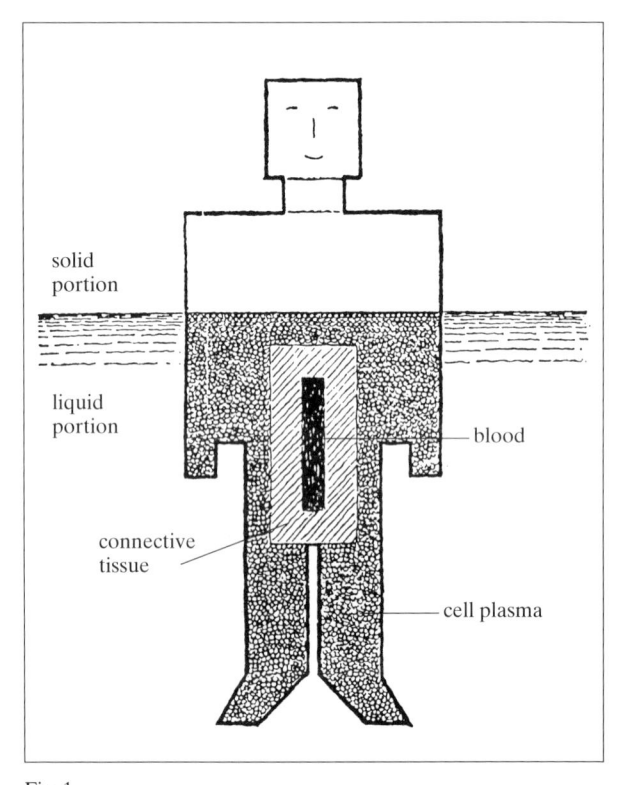

Fig. 1

substances that are transported in the blood must pass through the connective tissue to reach the cells. Waste products formed during combustion must also pass through the connective tissue in order to be removed by the blood. This is an important fact and it is crucial to the understanding of how MLD works.

3.2 Circulation

The left side of the heart pumps oxygen-rich blood through arteries, which branch into smaller arteries, which further branch into arterioles and these into capillaries. In order to be able to understand capillary function better, we subdivide them into an arterial and a venous loop. From the venous part of the capillary the blood flows into venules, from there into small, then large veins. First-order veins bring the blood to the right side of the heart, the starting point of the pulmonary circulation, i.e. arteries transport the oxygen-poor blood to the pulmonary alveoli (capillaries), where CO_2 is released and O_2 taken up. The oxygen-rich blood is then conveyed to the left side of the heart by veins. From there it is again pumped to the capillaries, where O_2 is unloaded from the transport vehicle haemoglobin, and CO_2 is loaded.

Strictly speaking, O_2 and haemoglobin become oxyhaemoglobin and this oxyhaemoglobin releases O_2 in the capillaries, which then diffuses into the tissue. On the other hand, CO_2 is transported as gas dissolved in the aqueous portion of the blood. Some of the CO_2 in the blood then reacts chemically with water as follows:

$CO_2 + H_2O$ produce H_2CO_3 or carbonic acid which dissociates to H and HCO_3. The receptors for the concentration of CO_2 in blood are in the carotid sinus and influence the breathing centre.

Parallel to the venous system, we have still another vessel system, the lymph system, so that one can say the arterial network is the supply system to the tissues and the venous and lymph networks the drainage systems. They have different tasks. The venous system, besides having the task of conducting the blood back to the heart, must also remove small molecular substances from the connective tissue and transport them. Small molecular substances include salts, sugars, water, and gases. They have a molecular weight of less than 200 – comparable to the head of a pin. The lymph system is responsible for removing large molecular substances and water from tissue and transporting them. Large molecular substances include protein molecules of various sizes. They have a molecular weight of 70,000 to 130,000 comparable to a boulder. A red blood corpuscle could be compared to an entire mountain. The lymph system can even remove the entire mountain, the blood corpuscle, from the tissue and transport it away. This explains the excellent results obtained in the treatment of blood effusions with MLD. These large molecular substances, which can only be removed from tissue via the lymph system, are designated lymph-obligatory load. This includes proteins, immobile cells, cell fragments, waste products, bacteria, viruses, inorganic substances, water and large-molecular fats.

3.3 Lymph system

Lymph vessels can be viewed with x-rays by filling them with a contrast-medium fluid. Blue dye bound to protein is injected subcutaneously. After a while a lateral incision is made in the skin between the injection site and the heart, and the vessels are exposed. Those vessels that are dyed blue are lymph vessels. These are now filled with contrast medium and can be radiologically displayed. The lymph vessels then usually look like strings of pearls. The constrictions are the valves, the pearls are the filled lymphatic segments [25]. Functional tests of the lymph vessels are performed using lymphoscintigraphic imaging.

3.4 Lymph nodes

Lymph nodes are included in the lymph paths as filtering stations [25]. As a rule, lymph does not leave an organ or a body region without undergoing filtering through a lymph node. Lymph nodes are connected to the circulatory system. They are made up of a connective tissue capsule, trabecula, marginal and intermediary sinuses, medulla, hilum and efferent and afferent lymph vessels as well as reticular tissue. Blood vessels enter the lymph nodes at the depression known as the hilum. Lymph entering by numerous afferent lymph vessels is concentrated in the lymph nodes. These vessels pierce the lymph node capsule from all sides. The lymph flows into the marginal sinus then into the cavities created by the trabecula (intermediary and medullary sinuses). It washes round the lymphocytes, plasma cells, and phagocytes, i.e. all the

Lymph nodes 3.4

cells of the immune system and leaves the node at the hilum via efferent lymph vessels. It should be pointed out that both B lymphocytes and T lymphocytes are found in the lymph nodes.

A lymphocyte that has been sensitised by an encounter with antigen is able to divide. In this way a defence system with a specific action is built up. Both the sensitised lymphocyte and its descendants are able to react specifically against this antigen and counteract it.

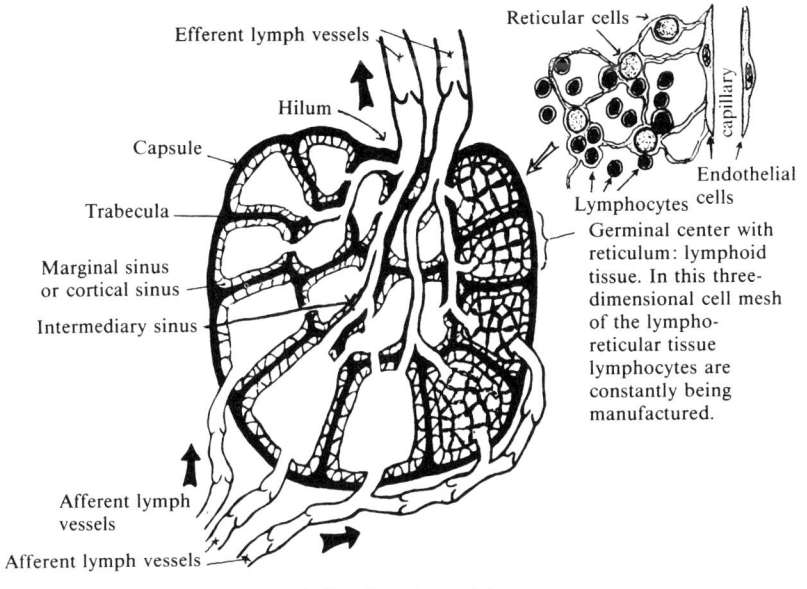

Fig. 2: Diagram of a lymph node (minus blood vessels)

Agglomerations of B lymphocytes in the lymph nodes are called lymph follicles. A distinction is made between primary follicles and the secondary follicles into which they develop in response to challenge by the infectious outside world. In completing their route through the body, the lymphocytes remain for some hours to some days in the lymph nodes but never more than 24 hours in the blood. The actual life of B lymphocytes is 3 to 8 days, that of T lymphocytes 100 to 150 days.

In the recognition of antigens the concept of self and nonself figures prominently. The feature self is embodied in all of the body's intact molecules, while the same molecule type produced in another individual is recognised as foreign because the spatial arrangement of its atoms is different. It is proteins that mediate the characteristic self or

3 Transport systems in the body

non-self feature. Thus viruses and bacteria, which are made up of protein, are combatted by our immune system as well as degenerate cells from our own body.

There are about 600 lymph nodes in the body, and some 160 in the neck region alone [23]. Lymph nodes not only bind, attack and breakdown antigens, but substances are also deposited there which the body cannot get rid of, e.g. glass dust, coal dust, mineral dust and dyes. The lymph is concentrated, which means its fluid is resorbed by blood capillaries.

The close resemblance of the reticular connective tissue to the embryonic mesenchyma explains, among other things, why surgically removed lymph nodes are able to regenerate completely from even small remaining capsule fragments. After total extirpation no regeneration takes place; also after induced chronic infections no new lymph nodes develop.

In the physiologic or accidental involution (retrograde change) of lymphatic organs the lymphoreticular tissue is increasingly replaced, beginning at the hilus, by fatty tissue and collagenous connective tissue. The lymph vessel system involutes especially in the mucous membranes, so that in old age it is absent in many areas.

Whether regular lymph drainage prevents or delays the involution of the lymph system is left to the reader's imagination. The fact is that proof is still lacking. After working 30 years with MLD, however, we have the impression the MLD does indeed bring improved function of the lymph system.

We know that organs which are in continuous use degenerate less than those which are used less or not at all. MLD ensures that the lymph vessel system is constantly exercised.

The majority of the organism's immunological reactions occur in the lymph nodes. One could also designate the lymph nodes as filtering stations which insure that only purified lymph reaches the blood. Otherwise our blood would become contaminated. In general the lymph nodes are devoid of musculature. There are, however, lymph nodes in the intestinal region which are provided with muscles and are therefore able to contract.

Summarizing, the functions of the lymph nodes are:
- Biological filter,
- Concentrating lymph. Strictly speaking, the lymph vessel walls are not completely watertight. Colloid osmotic pressure from neigh-

bouring veins exerts an influence through the lymph vessel walls. Water is reabsorbed into the veins, which results in a *thickening* of the lymph.
- Immunological function (replication of lymphocytes),
- Storage (for substances that are not broken down and cannot be removed such as coal dust etc.).

3.5 Anatomy of the lymph vessels

The largest lymph vessel in the human body is the thoracic duct. It originates in the cisterna chyli, a large lymph cistern in the navel region, and ascends through the diaphragm in front of the vertebral column. At the level of the sternoclavicular joint it arches to the left and empties into the left subclavian vein at the venous arch.

It transports the lymph of the lower body and legs (the watershed is the navel, 2nd lumbar vertebra). It also takes up some of the lymph generated in the thorax.

With precisely executed Manual Lymph Drainage, we can influence the lymph vessels of the skin. Thus, it is important to know the direction of drainage in order to apply appropriate lymph drainage. The body's covering (skin) is subdivided by watersheds into a number of territories. The body is divided into an **upper** and **lower half** (which includes the legs) by a great watershed which proceeds along the navel, iliac crest and the 2nd lumbar vertebra. The large lymph nodes of the **lower body** are the inguinal lymph nodes, which drain off the lymph from the legs. Lymph vessels from the soles of the feet, achilles tendon and calf musculature empty their contents into the popliteal lymph nodes (hollow of the knee). From there, the vessels proceed along the femur to the deep-seated lymph nodes in the groin. Instep, shin, lower leg skin and the entire thigh likewise go into the inguinal lymph nodes. There, one finds superficial (epifascial) and deep-seated (subfascial) lymph nodes which are connected with one another. The lymph vessels of the legs are unusual in that they are what is known as long vessels. Then there are what are known as physiological bottlenecks on the medial side of the ankle and knee. The lymph of the abdominal skin and buttocks, as well as the external genitalia and the scrotal skin likewise drain into the inguinal lymph nodes. From there, the lymph tracts proceed through the inguinal ligament on into the true pelvis, where the iliac node group receives the lymph of the urogenital organs (e.g. bladder, prostate).

3 Transport systems in the body

From the true pelvis, the vessels proceed along the aorta and the inferior vena cava to the Cisterna chyli. The lumbar lymph tracts are found arranged as a plexus (network). They drain the lymph of the kidneys, testicles, ovaries, oviduct and uterus. The coeliac trunk gathers the lymph of the spleen, pancreas, stomach, duodenum, gallbladder and the lower part of the liver. The intestinal trunk receives the lymph of the intestinal convolution, especially long-chain fat molecules from the digestive tract. (Short-chain fatty acids are carried via portal circulation directly to the liver.) All of these vessels proceed on to the Cisterna chyli – or take part in forming it – from which the thoracic duct originates. The liver capsule and the convex side of the liver are an exception in the abdominal region: the lymph from these flows in its own vessels through the diaphragm to the right lymphatic duct.

Thus it can be said that all lymph originating below the navel is transported by the thoracic duct.

Upper body: The lymph outflows of the upper body are also subdivided into lymph pathways of the skin and lymph vessels which drain the organs. The large lymph nodes of the upper body are the axillary lymph nodes. The upper body is subdivided into quadrants based on watersheds. There is a vertical watershed which extends from the jugular fossa to the symphysis; another watershed exists alongside the spinal column. There are watersheds running along the clavicle and the spine of the scapula. This results in 4 quadrants for the upper body skin, each draining into the corresponding axillary lymph nodes. The lymph from the arms flows via a mid-station (lymph nodes) in the elbow and the medial bicipital groove on to the axillary lymph nodes. The muscles are drained via large lymph vessels alongside the humerus. From the axillary lymph nodes, the subclavian trunk proceeds under and through the M. pectoralis major, bringing the lymph to its corresponding terminus. The lymph pathways of the arm can take a number of directions. The lymph vessels of the subcutis of the arm possess numerous anastomoses which connect the lymph pathways with each other, unlike the lymph vessels of the legs, as described above. From the radial catchment area (thumb and index finger), lymph vessels proceed along the cephalic vein via infraclavicular lymph nodes directly to the venous arch. The lateral part of the upper arm is likewise drained into these lymph nodes. The intercostal lymph tracts, which drain the intercostal spaces, flow along the anterior side of the thorax to the parasternal vessels. The intercostal spaces of the back drain into the thoracic duct. In the case of the intercostal spaces, which drain parasternally, there are descending and ascending lymph pathways, so that the lymph is drained, on the one hand, to the terminus, or else through the diaphragm into the Cisterna chyli. There are numerous anastomoses between the lymph pathways of the intercostal musculature and the skin of the thorax. Lymph from the thoracic organs is drained by three large lymph trunks both on the right and left sides. These are the bronchomediastinal, parasternal and anterior mediastinal trunks. Exceptions in the thoracic cavity are the heart and the lower left lobe of the lung, both of which are drained, along with the right lobe of the lung, via the right mediastinalis trunk. The mammary gland can be divided into 4 quadrants: the lymph of the lateral quadrants flows to the axilla; the medial upper quadrant drains parasternal to the terminus; the medial lower quadrant drains into the Cisterna chyli. The nipple drains into all four quadrants, so the division into quadrants should not be viewed too strictly.

The lymph of the skin and muscles of the head and neck is taken by the jugular trunk to the venous arch of that side. There are many anastomoses in the neck and facial region. The cervical lymph nodes are situated epifascially and subfascially in the tissue. In addition, the brain's lymph-obligatory load flows through the lymph nodes of the neck. The brain and spinal cord have no lymph vessels: the pre-lymph from this area drains via the cerebrospinal fluid (and other routes, e.g. along the spinal nerves). This is discussed in more detail in the advanced courses.

3.6 Summary of transport systems in the body

Substances in the body are transported rapidly over long distances via pipelines: blood vessels and lymph vessels. The blood is driven by the main pump, the heart; the lymph by auxiliary pumps, the musculature of the lymph vessels, the pressure difference created in the thorax by breathing, the movement of the skeletal muscles, peristaltic movement of the intestine, and pulsation of the arteries. The transport of substances in connective tissue is accomplished by diffusion.

3 Transport systems in the body

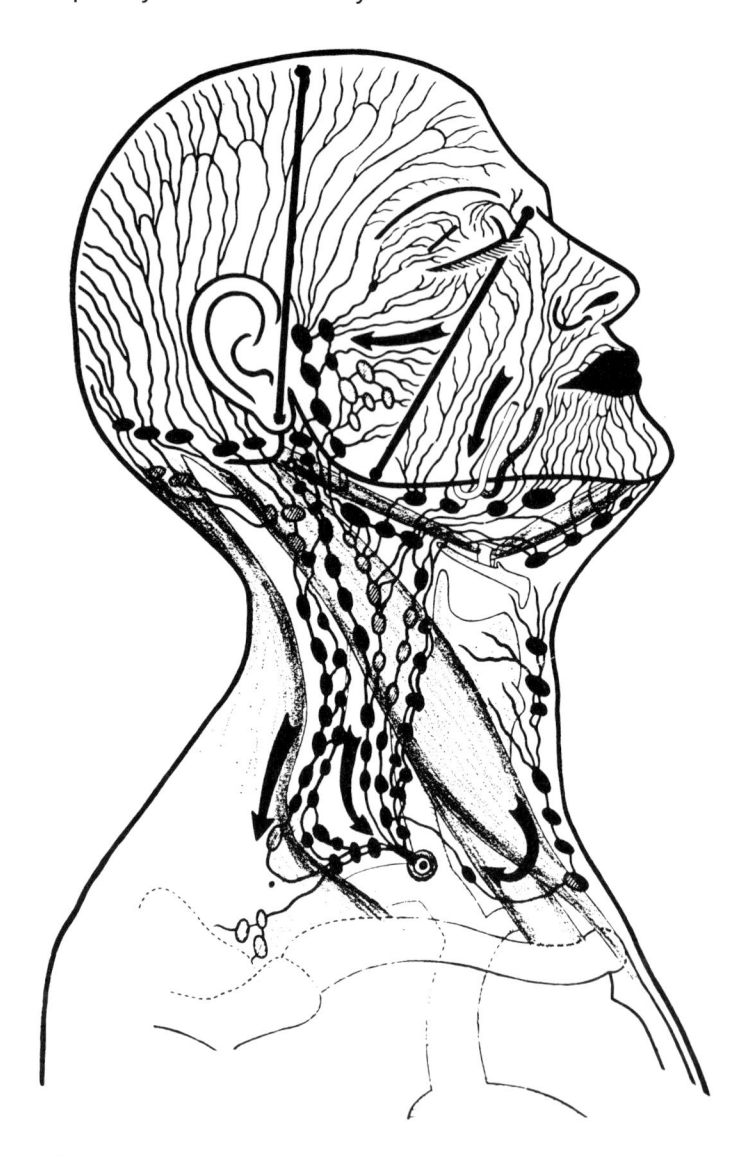

Fig. 3

Summary of transport systems in the body 3.6

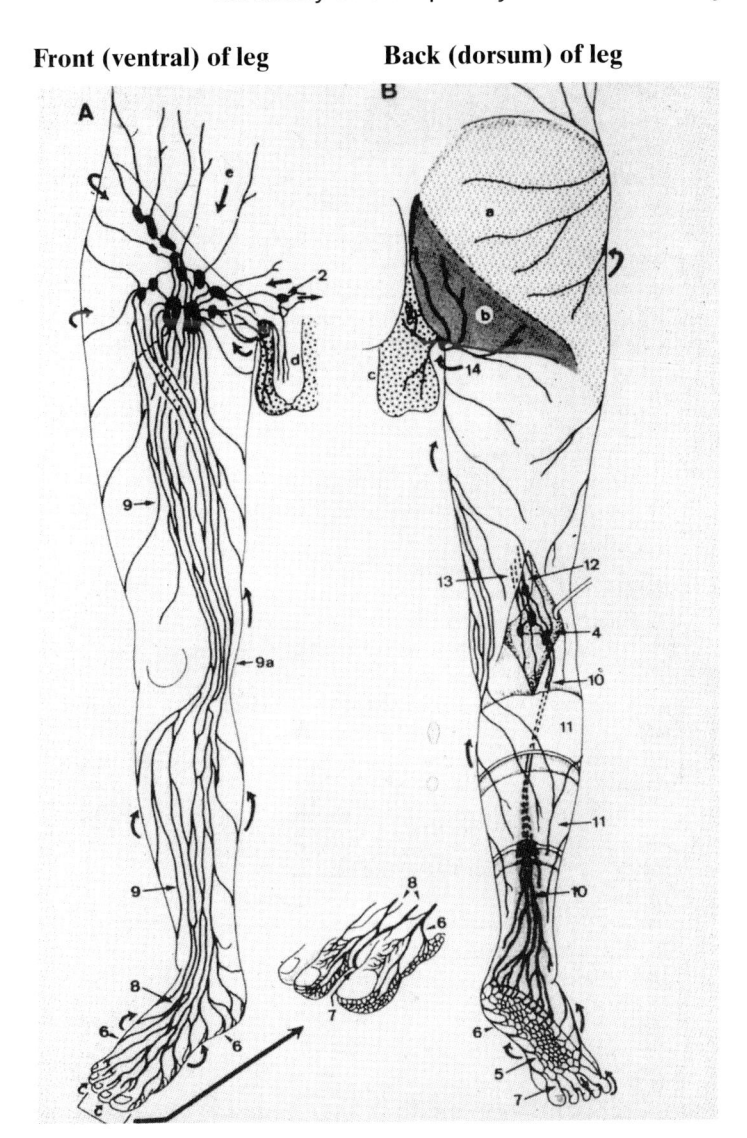

Front (ventral) of leg **Back (dorsum) of leg**

Fig. 4: Catchment area of the superficial inguinal and popliteal lymph nodes.
1) superficial inguinal lymph nodes, 2) prepubic lymph nodes, 3) lymph nodes of the penis, 4) popliteal lymph nodes, 5) plantar lymph plexus, 6) medial plantar vessels, 7) interdigital plantar vessels, 8) collectors of the dorsum of the foot, 9) ventromedial bundle, 9a) popliteal section of the ventromedial bundle: physiological bottleneck, 10) dorsolateral bundle, 11) superficial cruris fascia, 12) adductor canal hiatus, 13) femoral lymph vessels, 14) genitofemoral sulcus, a,b) gluteal region, c) perineum anus, scrotum, d) external genitalia, e) front abdominal wall, f) back

3 Transport systems in the body

Arm and Breast

1. Thoracic duct
2. Supraclavicular lymph nodes
3. Subclavian trunk
4. Infraclavicular lymph nodes
5. Interpectoral lymph nodes
6. Thoracoacromial lymph nodes
7. Central axillary lymph nodes
8. Lateral axillary lymph nodes
9. Brachial artery and vein
10. Radial bundle along the cephalic vein
11. Ulnar bundle along the cephalic vein
12. Profound cubital lymph nodes
13. Superficial cubital lymph nodes
14. Pectoral lymph nodes
15. Subscapular lymph nodes
16. Parasternal lymph nodes

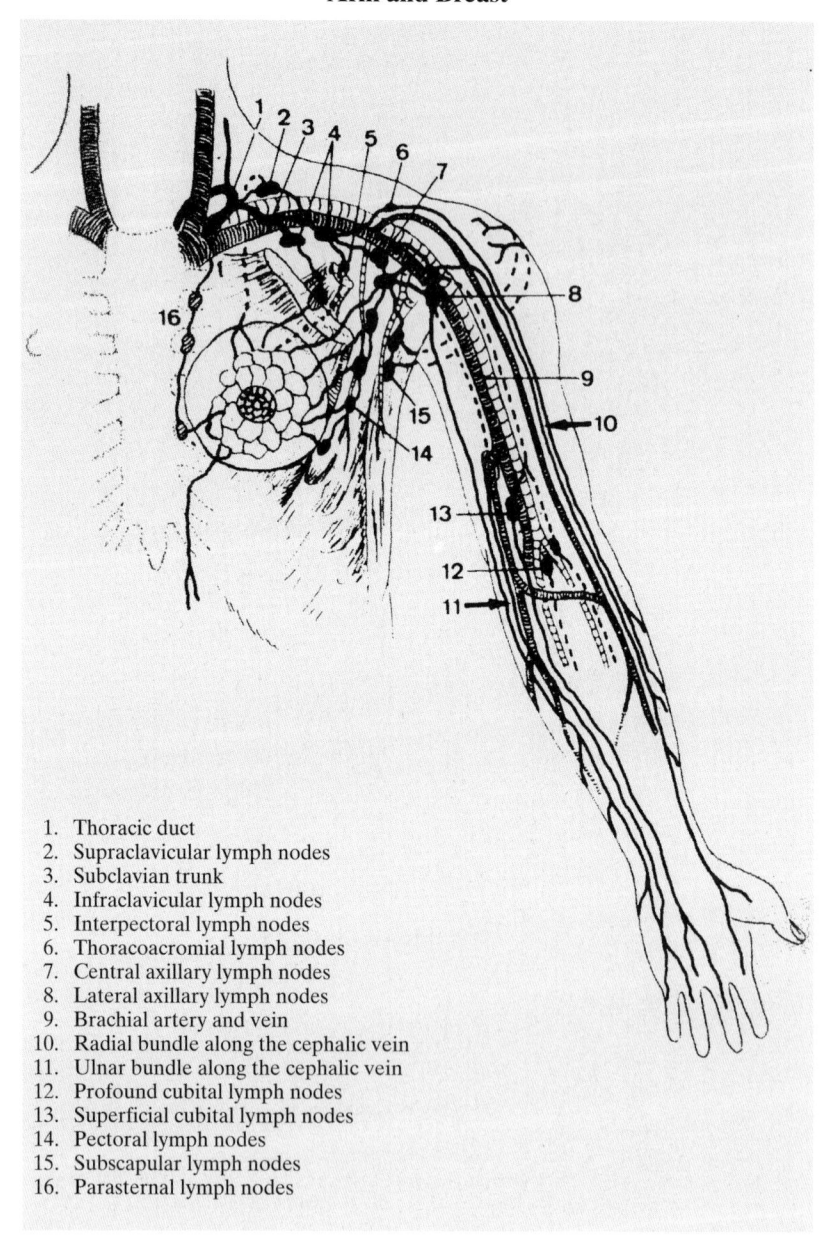

Fig. 5

Summary of transport systems in the body 3.6

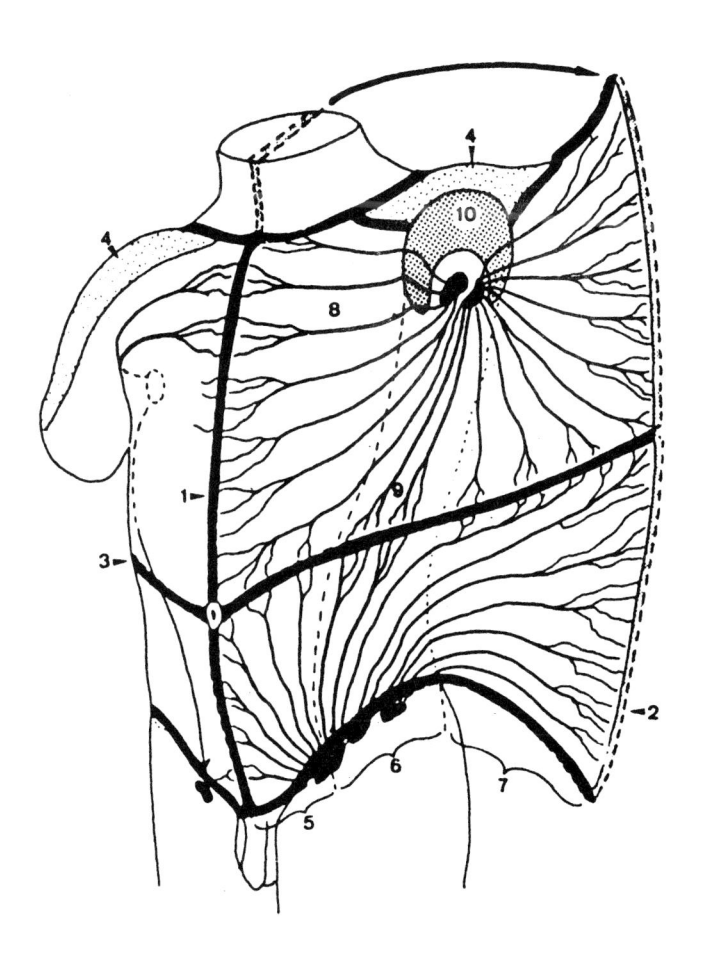

Fig. 6: Schematic representation of lymph drainage of the trunk wall (skin of back folded out). 1) Front vertical watershed, 2) rear vertical watershed, 3) transversal watershed, 4) drainage area of the lateral upper arm fascicle, 5) front trunk wall, 6) side trunk wall 7) rear trunk wall, 8) interaxillary collaterals, 9) axilloinguinal collaterals, 10) amputation site of shoulder.

3 Transport systems in the body

Main lymph trunks and lymph node groups in the body

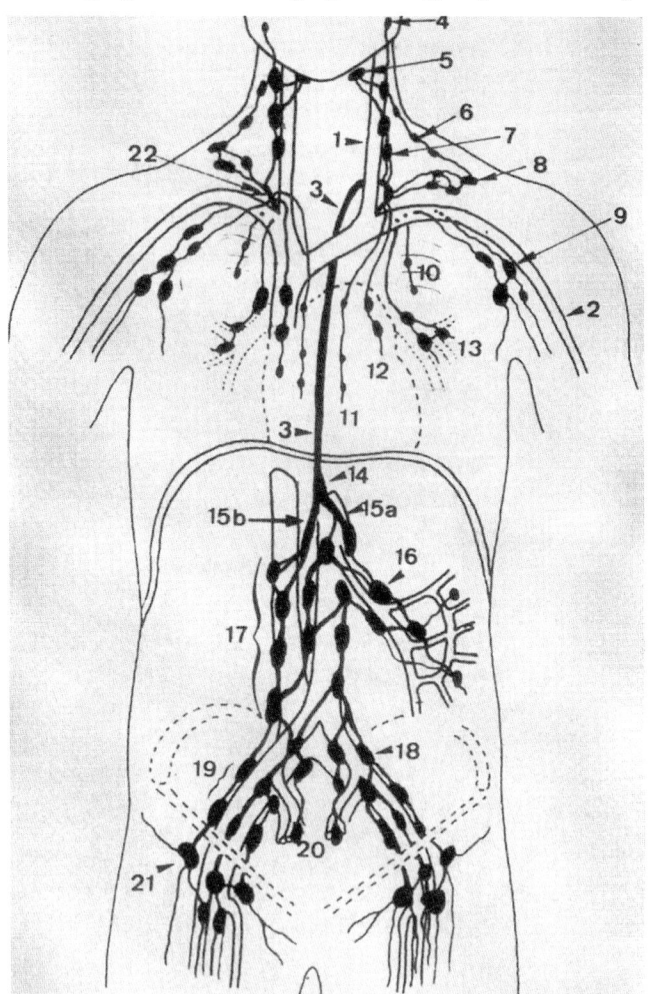

Fig. 7: 1) internal jugular vein (left), 2) subclavian vein (left), 3) thoracic duct, 4) parotid lymph nodes, 5) submandibular lymph nodes, 6) comittant accessory lymph nodes, 7) internal jugular lymph nodes with jugular trunk (left), 8) supraclavicular lymph nodes and trunk (left), 9) axillary lymph nodes with subclavian trunk (left), 10) intercostal lymph nodes with intercostal trunk (left), 11) parasternal lymph nodes with parasternal trunk (left), 12) anterior mediastinal lymph nodes with anterior mediastinal trunk (left), 13) tracheobronchial lymph nodes with tracheobronchial trunk (left), 14) Cystema chyli, 15a) left lumbar trunk, 15b) right lumbar trunk, 16) mesenteric lymph nodes, 17) lumbar lymph nodes, 18) iliac lymph nodes, 19) iliac lymph nodes, 20) iliac lymph nodes, 21) inguinal lymph nodes.

4 Substance transport

4.1 Molecular motion

Every molecule is in motion, owing to the thermal energy it contains. This motion would cease at absolute zero (–273° C or 0 Kelvin). For example, the wood molecules in a table top vibrate in place. Molecules of a fluid or gas move in a straight path until they collide with other molecules of the same type. They then ricochet like billiard balls, collide again, and thereby change their position. This spontaneous movement of molecules give rise to diffusion, provided that a concentration gradient exists. If this is not the case, the molecules will still move, but then the process is no longer diffusion, which is a transport mechanism.

4.2 Diffusion [14]

The molecules of a lump of sugar dissolving in the bottom of a coffee cup are in motion, colliding with and rebounding off each other, some entering the sugar-free part of the coffee, so that eventually the sugar and coffee are mixed together. The process of this sugar migration is called diffusion. After 4-6 weeks, the sugar would be uniformly distributed throughout the coffee. We therefore see that diffusion strives towards a concentration equilibrium or one could also say, diffusion moves in the direction of lower concentration. Strictly speaking, this is only a generalization. Some of the molecules, through collision, also move in the direction of higher concentration. Statistically, however, the majority of molecules move in the direction of lower concentration as a result of random collisions. Diffusion is also temperature-dependent, i.e. the colder the milieu, the slower the diffusion; the warmer the milieu, the faster the diffusion. Large molecules move slower than small molecules. The time of diffusion increases as the square of the distance. Therefore diffusion requires short distances if it is to effectively exercise its transport function.

If the diffusion distance exceeds 1 nm (nanometre) diffusion becomes questionable as a means of transport, because, for example, it would require an hour to cover 1.3 mm. On the other hand it takes only one third of a second to travel 0.01 nm, the diameter of a large cell.

4.3 Substance transport in the connective tissue

An oxygen molecule entering the body through the lungs is bound to hemoglobin in the alveoli and transported by the blood stream. It is unloaded in a capillary. The oxygen concentration in capillaries is high, since oxygen is unloaded there, whereas the oxygen concentration in the cell is low because cells burn O_2. The migration of O_2 from the capillary to the cell and of CO_2 from the cell to the capillary proceeds according to the principles of diffusion. Like gases transported in tissue, food and vital substances for the cells are also subject to the laws of diffusion. The same applies for waste products of cellular combustion, which are taken up by the capillaries and transported in the bloodstream to the excretory organs.

4.4 Osmosis

In order to fully understand the transport processes at the capillary, i.e. diffusion, filtration and resorption, we need to explain the term osmosis.

Osmosis is diffusion through a semipermeable membrane. If this membrane separates two solutions of differing concentrations e.g. water and saltwater, then the two solutions have different *water concentrations*. The side containing salt has less water molecules. The other side strives for a concentration equilibrium and water molecules diffuse through the membrane towards the salt side. The increase in pressure is called the osmotic pressure of the fluid. Osmosis is the water-attracting force of salt and sugar whereas oncosis is the ability of proteins to take up water.

5 Effect of MLD on blood capillaries and connective tissue

5.1 Structure and function of blood capillaries

The blood capillaries show differences in their wall structure, depending on the organ in which they are located. In other words, the capillaries are organ-specific in their construction. Thus there are regions in which the capillaries are more or less impermeable. There are also fenestrated capillaries or [7] simple porous basement membrane tubes that are lined on the inside with a layer of endothelial cells and coated on the outside with a layer of pericytes cells with diameters of 5–10 µ (5–10/1000 mm). Blood capillaries are sometimes narrower than an erythrocyte, which must therefore deform itself to be able to pass through. The basement membrane is made of interwoven collagen fibrils embedded in an amorphous ground substance. The collagen fibrils are not very tightly interwoven; they have gaps measuring 30 to 45 Å – occasionally up to 100 Å. The basement membrane separates at places to enclose a pericyte (they are often noticeable in the brain but in contrast are totally absent in skeletal muscle). Pericytes contain the same organelles as endothelial cells, including abundant pinocytic vesicles. The healthy basement membrane is 300–800 Å thick. One capillary is approximately 1 mm long, and all capillaries laid end to end would measure 200,000 km – more than half the distance from the earth to the moon. Osmosis takes place through the capillary pores. An estimated 70,000 litres of water diffuse through the capillary walls every day. This amount of water is possible only because we have an astronomical number of capillaries in our body. According to Wendt, capillary basement membranes, and in more extreme cases the intima of the arterioles as well, represent a reservoir for excess dietary protein, since they thicken as they accumulate surplus protein. This constitutes a barrier to osmosis and thus to cell nourishment and the removal of waste products from the cells.

A capillary combines two opposing characteristics. It must be leak-proof, so that blood can flow through it and it must be permeable, so that substances can diffuse through its pores. Water and nutrients reach tissue via the capillary wall not only by osmosis, but also by filtration. An estimated 70 litres of water – 1000 times less than through diffusion

5 Effect of MLD on blood capillaries and connective tissue

– is filtered daily through capillary walls. Blood capillary pressure is the driving force behind filtration and the amount of filtrate is determined by the blood pressure in the capillary. At the same time, other forces are operative which will be described later in the text.

Resorption is part of capillary **filtration**. Its function is to resorb the filtered water back into the capillary. The force that powers resorption is contained in the blood proteins which collect water by means of a special type of suction pressure known as oncotic pressure or colloid osmotic pressure. The average protein content of the blood is approximately 7.4%. These proteins are able to resorb the water filtered at normal blood pressure, so that a fluid equilibrium (Starling equilibrium) is maintained in the pericapillary spaces. Thus, a flow of liquid through the capillary is brought about by filtration and resorption which occurs independently of diffusion. Filtration is a flow of liquid through the capillary wall into the connective tissue, where it is reclaimed via the oncotic suction (colloid-osmotic pressure) of the blood proteins.

5.2 The Starling Equilibrium

Starling described in 1897 the four forces which act on the capillaries:

1. Blood capillary pressure and colloid-osmotic pressure (oncotic suction) of the tissue as filtration forces.
2. Tissue pressure and colloid-osmotic pressure (oncotic suction) of the blood as resorption forces.

Under physiologic conditions a fluid equilibrium prevails at the terminal vessels. This means that the hydrostatic capillary pressure filters fluid into tissue, while the colloid osmotic pressure of the blood again resorbs the fluid. Starling himself did not express his hypothesis as a mathematical formula.

This Starling's Law only has statistical significance as it doesn't take into account that blood capillaries in most regions of the body are not permeable to protein. Proteins can generally only leave the tissues via the lymph pathways. Thus, wherever there is protein permeation, oedema should arise. However, an oedema only occurs when lymph drainage is disturbed (see oedema). The permeability of the capillaries for protein is regionally different, as well as protein passage in the venules by means of cytopempis or as a result of permeability of the venule walls. A functional lymph drainage is therefore necessary to maintain the fluid equilibrium. Dr. Vodder's Lymph Drainage stimulates lymph flow, because its special manipulations accelerate the contraction of the lymph segments. The subcutaneous lymph vessels are interlinked in a network. With the manual acceleration of the lymph flow there is an increase in the lymph flow of the entire region. This is associated with a suction action, which eventually exerts an effect in the soft connective tissue.

5.3 Effect of MLD via the blood capillaries and lymph vessels

At first, only stimulation of lymph flow was ascribed to Dr. Vodder's method of Manual Lymph Drainage. It was assumed that MLD drained oedematous tissue only through the lymph vessels. Scientific experiments were carried out on rats [5,16] in order to prove this. Lymphostatic oedema was artificially induced and then treated with MLD. The results were striking. The oedema was almost entirely drained from the tissue by the action of MLD. The control group, on the contrary, had severe oedema. The oedema was drained from the tissue even though the lymph vessels leading away from the tissue had been tied off. These findings raised new questions. How and through what means could the oedema have been drained if not through the lymph vessels?

Two possibilities arose: that the water was removed from the tissues via the blood capillaries and/or, as we now know, that lymph was shifted via the valveless initial lymph vessels that lie in the subpapillary layer of the skin (Kubik's *lymphatic areas*) to functional lymph vessels.

As far as tissue fluid is concerned MLD has two effective directions. First, the appropriate massage pressure has the same effect as an elastic bandage or the hydrostatic pressure in hydrotherapy, i.e. a resorptive effect. The net ultrafiltrate is thus reduced. The acceleration of blood flow in the capillaries, established by Curri [46], leads to the conclusion that reabsorption is elevated.

The second draining effect of MLD occurs via the valveless initial lymph vessels as mentioned earlier. Besides water, it is possible to take protein out of the tissues as part of the lymph-obligatory load by stimulating the lymphangio-motoricity. This is how we have a flushing effect of MLD on the lymph-obligatory load. It is obvious that the massage

5 Effect of MLD on blood capillaries and connective tissue

pressure applied will have a decisive influence on this effect. MLD especially differs from classical massage in that less pressure is used.

Salts can have the same water-binding effect as proteins in the connective tissue. Mucopolysaccharides should also not be forgotten. These large molecules can store water and protein. It is not certain whether MLD also has an effect on these bound substances – water and protein, and at best only surmised.

6 The significance of optimal massage pressure

In MLD treatment the optimal massage pressure is the pressure that achieves the best possible results. Thus, it is the pressure that removes the greatest possible amount of water as well as protein from the tissue. A closer look, however, reveals that a given effect is accounted for not only by the massage pressure, but also by the way in which the pressure is applied.

In the original Dr. Vodder method specific receptors are stimulated that ensure optimal tissue drainage [27]. Since the condition of the patients' tissues varies widely, both the pressure and technique must be adapted to the findings. This optimal massage can only be learned under the supervision of a lymph drainage teacher with many years of practical experience in treating patients. The range of MLD techniques is very broad and correct pressure can only be learned by repeated comparison between the student and the teacher. A definite upper pressure limit is marked by the occurrence of pain. Whenever MLD causes pain, you may be assured that it is being applied incorrectly. A reddening of the skin should be avoided if possible. MLD is classified within the broad framework of classical massage and is one of the large-area, soft massage methods with a special technique that brings about a pumping action in the tissue.

7 Inertial Mass

In order to understand MLD, the term inertial mass must be explained. Honey for example, is an inertial mass. If a coin is dropped into honey it takes a time to disappear into this inertial mass.

A broken-down car is an inertial mass. What can we do to move it? It can be pushed, i.e. energy is applied to this inertial mass to move it. We can do this in two ways: we can take a running start at the car though we know the inertial mass will not move. We can however apply energy by leaning or pressing against the car, though this will take more time. Now the inertial mass begins to move. These examples show that apart from energy, time is also needed to move the inertial mass.

Connective tissue, as well as lymphoedema, reacts like an inertial mass. This explains the long treatment times allowed during MLD. Our experience has shown that the longer the treatment takes the greater the success of treatment with MLD will be. This shows that the greater the inertial mass (more fluid in the tissue), the slower and longer the techniques have to be applied if the fluid in the tissues is to be moved.

8 Steel and rubber elasticity

To demonstrate steel and rubber elasticity, imagine a T bar with a steel spring on one side and a rubber band on the other. If successive weights of equal size are added to the steel spring it will stretch accordingly by equal distances. If they are then removed one by one, the spring returns in equal steps to its original size. Thus a steel spring stretches proportionately to its original size. This steel elastic behaviour is shown by collagen fibres.

In contrast the rubber band stretches a lot with the first weight, less so with the second and even less with the third weight, even though the weights are equal. Thus it stretches disproportionately with the weight applied. If the weight is removed after a certain time then the rubber band doesn't return to its original position because rubber is subject to stretching and aging processes.

The phenomenon is that this rubber band gradually shrinks to its original position, a process called **hysteresis**. This process is dependent on the age of the rubber and the duration of the stretching. Elastic fibres also have this typical rubber elastic behaviour.

This is of the greatest importance to all those practicing Manual Lymph Drainage. Oedematous tissue that has been drained of excess fluid using MLD does not return to its original position. In a sense it has been deformed. By using external support bandages or elastic stockings, we enhance our treatment and ensure success treating such tissues. We thereby prevent fluid returning to the tissues and promote the hysteresis.

9 The lymph vessel system

Taken from:
FOLIA ANGIOLOGICA/Vol. XXVIII/7/8/9/80
St. Kubik: Drainage possibilities of the lymph territories

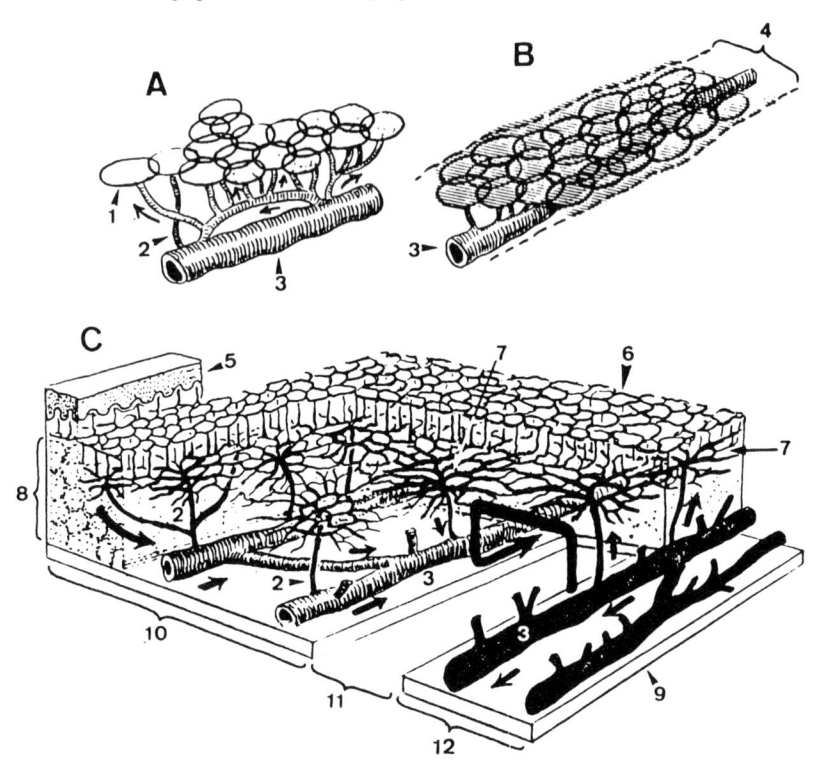

Fig. 8: Schematic representation of lymph drainage of the skin.
A) areas, B) lymphatic skin zones, C) drainage pathways of congested areas, 1) skin areas, 2) precollector, 3) subcutaneous collector, 4) lymphatic skin zone, 5) skin, 6) superficial cutaneous layer, 7) deep cutaneous rete, 8) subcutis, 9) fascia, 10) normal lymph territory, 11) lymphatic watershed, 12) congested territory.

9.1 Lymphatic watersheds [31, 47]

The superficial drainage system is divided into lymphatic areas and territories, depending on the size of the drainage paths. The overlapping skin areas (valveless, initial lymph vessels in the subpapillary layer of the skin) are drained by valved precollectors. The valves of the precollectors protect the initial network from backward filling. The overlapping of skin areas permits drainage in every direction. The precollectors of several skin areas usually join with a trunk collector of the subcutis. The skin areas of one collector form a type of striped skin zone. The skin zones are connected with each other by anastomoses in the cutaneous lymph vessel network and above all, by many connections with neighbouring collectors. According to Kubik, the skin zones of all the collectors of a lymph vessel bundle form a territory. The borders of a territory are known as lymphatic watersheds and there are no collectors to connect the territories. If the collectors are imagined as a net, the net begins at a watershed. Another network begins on the other side of this watershed which drains in a different direction. Normally lymph does not flow over the watershed because the resistance to flow in this direction is greater than the direction of flow of the territorial collectors in the subcutis.

These two drainage territories separated at the level of the collectors are nevertheless interconnected. Since the skin regions anastomose with each other, it is possible in pathological cases to drain lymph from one territory, over a watershed to another territory by means of MLD. This is via the precollectors and valveless cutaneous vessels. The subcutaneous layer of the skin is usually affected in oedema. This is why it is important to influence the superficial lymph vessels which drain the skin and subcutis.

These watersheds drawn by Kubik largely agree with those of Sappey. Since Sappey's drawings helped Dr. Vodder to develop and specify his manipulations for the manual drainage of the lymph territories, no improvement was necessary when Kubik published his anatomic work on the lymph vessel system of human skin. More evidence of the acumen with which Dr. Vodder developed Manual Lymph Drainage.

9.2 Anatomy and function of the initial lymph vessels

The more protein found in the tissues, the less water can flow out of the tissues via the blood capillaries because protein binds water. The lymph vessel system is then responsible for transporting water out of the tissue together with protein so that water can again flow out via the blood capillaries [14]. The initial lymph vessels begin blind in the tissues like the fingers of a glove. They are joined by filaments to the collagen fibres of the connective tissue. The free margins of the endothelial cells overlap and can flap about, i.e. they move inward and outward. In this sense, one can speak of flap valves. Now if the connective tissue swells due to an increased influx of water, the pressure rises. The collagen fibres are separated from each other and pull the filaments (fibre mat) fixed to the endothelial cells with them. Openings appear in the initial lymph vessels, through which water and large molecular substances can enter the lumen of the vessel. Large cells such as erythrocytes can also enter the initial lymph vessel in this way. As a result of the modified pressure relationships created by the filling of the initial lymph vessel (the connective tissue pressure decreases due to eflux of water and the internal pressure of the initial lymph vessel increases), the flap valves close. The initial lymph vessel is now full and sealed. The filaments return to their original positions since the amount of water in the connective tissue has decreased.

Recent research confirms that the initial lymph vessel has a basal membrane consisting of fine reticular fibres. This felt-like *fibre mat* is connected with the connective tissue fibers. Large molecules or cells seek out small openings – usually smaller than a cell diameter – in the fibre mat and then advance through an open junction in the endothelial cells into the lumen of the initial lymph vessel.

A recent publication by Tischendorf [25] and a personal discussion describes the action of initial lymph vessels as follows:

Some of the initial lymph vessel endothelial cells are arranged in such a way that they appear folded or overlapping. Also present are adjacent endothelial cells bound together by hyaluronic acid cement. The protein molecules diffusing into the initial lymph vessel open these cemented joints by pushing hyaluronidase in front of them. Hyaluronidase liquefies (depolymerizes) hyaluronic acid cement and the protein slips into the initial lymph vessel. The cement resolidifies afterwards. This hyaluronic acid-hyaluronidase interaction occurs continuously in the connective tissue.

From this viewpoint diffusion regulates the migration direction of protein and the rest of the lymph-obligatory load. A proximal emptying of the lymph vessels, e.g. through MLD, would thus increase the diffusion pressure in connective tissue by promoting vascular lymph flow and thus ultimately removing protein and the remaining lymph-obligatory load from the initial lymph vessel [28]. This proximal lymph drainage or emptying of the initial lymph vessels would also have the effect of lowering the pressure inside the initial lymph vessels. This means that

Anatomy and function of the initial lymph vessels 9.2

the existing difference between blood, interstitial and lymphatic pressures would increase. According to Bargmann, intercellular filtration into the initial lymph vessels follows immediately.

In Folia angiologica 7/8/9/80, G. Hauck describes prelymphatic tissue spaces and channels (also Casley-Smith, 1976), which are located in the connective tissue space and have the function of transporting proteins from the bloodstream relatively quickly to the initial lymph vessels. He observed that the elastic fibres of the connective tissue serve as guide rails for fluid transport. The rate of fluid transport is higher along the elastic fibres than by diffusion. The diameter of these channels is smaller than that of the initial lymph vessels and they eventually show a microscopically discernible wall structure. The beginning of wall formation is visible under light microscopy and evaluated as the site of a continuous transition into the lymph vessel system. These results permit the interpretation of the lymph system as a converging drainage system that is completely open in the periphery.

The function of the initial lymph vessel is lymph formation. By *lymph formation* we mean the influx of the lymph-obligatory load from the connective tissue into the initial lymph vessel. Currently, 5 possibilities are given to explain the mechanism of lymph formation:

1. Colloid-osmotic and hydrostatic pressure outside of and in the initial lymph vessels.
2. Mechanical pressure differentials.
3. Prelymphatic channels.
4. Histomechanical causes.
5. Suction exerted from precollectors and for collectors.

How does lymph get from the initial lymph vessel into the lymphangion?

Due to the increased internal pressure of the lymph capillaries, the *outlet valve* opens and the lymph pours into a precollector, the connection between the initial lymph vessels and the collectors of the subcutis. A contracting skeletal muscle can also exert pressure on a full vessel an accelerate its emptying.

Once the lymph is in the first lymphangion, it is then compressed by the contracting smooth muscle and thus pumped along from angion to angion. The formation of lymph is thus dependent on the connective

9 The lymph vessel system

tissue fluid volume, and is initiated if the blood capillaries cannot remove water from the connective tissue, i.e. if the tissue pressure rises. In such cases however, the lymph vessel system is capable of removing as much as 10 times more fluid than it normally does. The generally accepted normal daily lymph volume is 2–3 liters.

All the substances that are not resorbed by the blood-vessel system are collectively called the lymph-obligatory load because the lymphatic system is then the only route available for normalizing the connective tissue composition.

Hyaluronidase is employed as a drug medium in medicine and as an agent for treating panniculosis in cosmetics. It is sold in creams, tablets, and ampules. As early as 1967 [11] it was evident that the enzyme of hyaluronic acid causes the filaments of the endothelial cells in the initial lymph vessels to rupture. Hyaluronic acid is the substance that cements the fine filaments to the endothelial cells and to the collagen fibres. It is foolish and destructive to use hyaluronidase. According to Földi, the connective tissue ground substance is altered through depolymerization of the mucopolysaccharides and the cemented joints of the filaments (as described above) are dissolved. The initial lymph vessels collapse as a result of tissue pressure if the filaments are loosened from their anchorage. Lymph production is thus made impossible.

9.3 Protein circulation and transport

In this context, large molecular substances are mostly protein molecules. If there is too much protein in the blood [22], e.g. after a protein-rich meal, the capillary endothelial and epithelial cells act as regulators to reestablish normal blood protein concentration. The endothelial cells have three mechanisms for removing protein – including immune proteins and antigens – from the bloodstream.

1. Since the highest protein concentration is in the blood, there is a constant stream of protein to the intercellular spaces. The smaller proteins (albumins) especially, seep through large pores in the capillaries and thus reach the connective tissue.

2. The active transport of proteins through the endothelial cells by means of pinocytic vesicles which is known as cytopempis.

    A large number of pinocytic vesicles are found in endothelial cells.

The transport mechanism is as follows: The endothelial cell membrane projects into the lumen of the blood vessel and takes up a protein molecule which it then 'encloses' in a vesicle.

The vesicle carries the protein like an elevator through the cell, puts it out on the other side and releases the protein. Protein is constantly being transported from the blood to the tissue by this method of cytopempis. The transport of other substances by an active process is known as pinocytosis.

3. In order for a protein equilibrium to occur in the blood, there must be a mechanism to accommodate the fluctuations in protein concentration. According to Wendt [24], this mechanism is lodged in the ability of the endothelial cells to take up protein from the blood and during a lowered protein intake, to return it. This maintains a constant blood protein level.

In the case of endothelial cell permeation via cytopempis the molecular structure of the transiting protein remains unchanged, whereas proteins entering the cell and permeating the endothelial cytoplasm usually undergo molecular change. The flow of transendothelial protein from the blood to the basement membrane is a physiological, active process of endothelial cells. They withdraw protein from the blood, transform it into insoluble mucopolysaccharides and deposit it on the basement membrane. D.L. Fry concluded from this (at the 12th Ciba Symposium in London) that the endothelial surface is extremely sensitive to events occurring in the blood flowing by. This sensitivity can be seen as a monitoring function of endothelial cells in relation to endogenous substances with elevated blood levels as well as to foreign substances, e.g. antigens.

The physiological protein flow from blood into tissue through the endothelial cells and basement membrane, proceeds in such a way that protein permeating into tissue from the blood interacts with the basement membrane while passing through it. This protein permeation decreases permeability of the vessel wall by thickening it. The basement membrane is displaced from inside towards the outside because endothelial cells withdraw protein from the blood, transform it into insoluble mucopolysaccharides, and deposit it on the basement membrane. The epithelial cells transform the protein into soluble tissue protein on the outer wall of the basement membrane and release it into the tissue. In this way, the basement membrane slowly moves from the inside towards the outside, carrying the proteins deposited on it. Wendt calls

9 The lymph vessel system

this process glacial transport. Extremely efficient endothelial and epithelial cells break down resorbed proteins completely. If the protein is foreign, it is transformed into euprotein and poured back into the blood or transformed into mucopolysaccharide and deposited on the basement membrane. Weaker endothelial and epithelial cells are often unable to breakdown and transform all of the protein. If there are antigen-antibody complexes, some of these are deposited unbuffered on the basement membrane, which then causes inflammation (capillaritis).

We therefore have a physiological protein reservoir in connective tissue and a protein reservoir in the basement membrane – primarily in pathological situations. If the storage causes the basement membrane to become thicker than 1400 Å, the condition is pathological and filtration and diffusion are impaired. The body's regulatory mechanisms are responsible for adequate nourishment of the cells. This is accomplished by increasing the blood pressure in order to reestablish normal filtration and diffusion despite thickened basement membranes. Thus the permeability for nutrients depends on the degree of swelling of the basement membrane.

Continuous resorption of excess protein finally overloads the basement-membrane protein reservoir. The proteins become congested in the blood. They are then resorbed by arterial endothelium and deposited subendothelial as collagen on the intima of the arteries. This is the pathogenesis of arteriosclerosis and its associated risks.

We would first of all like to distinguish between **physiological** and **pathological** protein and food storage [22].

1. After healthy people eat a well-balanced meal, the blood levels of all the nutrient molecules are elevated. Reduction of the elevated nutrient levels to normal is achieved through the high diffusion pressures created by the elevated nutrient blood levels, which drive the nutrient molecules through the pores of the blood-capillary basement membrane into the connective-tissue. All the different types of nutrients are thus stored in the connective tissue, each in a storage molecule: protein in collagen and the amino groups of mucopolysaccharides, glucose in the sugar part of mucopolysaccharides, fat in fat cells, and excess water in the domain of the mucopolysaccharide molecules. The subcutaneous connective tissue of an overfed person may in this way become several centimetres thick. The voluminous connective tissue reservoir in overweight people is not only crammed with fatty tissue, but with all the other nutrients too, their

relative proportions depending on the nature of the diet that has led to the overweight condition.

As long as the capillary basement membranes are healthy, their pores open and the transport routes clear, all nutrients enter the connective tissue for cell nourishment or for storage. Thus the overfed person becomes overweight but remains healthy because an increase in connective tissue storage molecules has no harmful consequences.

2. Nutrient storage, especially protein storage, may become pathological, from eating too much food rich in animal protein. The basal membrane becomes thicker as a consequence of protein deposition; this increasingly impedes passage through the basal membrane of protein and all other nutrients, resulting in a sieve effect. (Sieve effect means that molecules cannot diffuse through the pores if a great number of these molecules appear at the capillary membrane at the same time. For example, if sand is shovelled into a sieve that is not in motion, the sand will remain in the sieve even though the grains are smaller than the holes in the sieve.)

According to Földi, all protein molecules leave the bloodstream within 24 to 48 hours. They enter the connective tissue and are for the most part transported back to the blood via the lymph vessel system, so that one can appropriately speak of protein circulation. To some extent, tissue protein also finds it way back into the blood via cytopempsis. The average diameter of a blood-capillary pore is 80-90 Å, occasionally up to 100 Å [7]. Albumin has a 70 Å diameter; a single molecule can pass through the large pores into the tissue. Gammaglobulins are larger than 100 Å. Albumin is a transport vehicle; it transports water, metals, enzymes, vitamins, penicillins, insulin, hormones. Gammaglobulins have defence functions; amino acids are the building blocks of proteins and therefore also of cells. Betaglobulins transport fat-like substances. All together there are over 100 different proteins in blood. Bennhold [18] describes a vehicular function of plasma proteins, transporting the vital substances to the cells and the metabolic wastes from them. The manifold duties of proteins show that protein circulation is no less important than any other circulation, and protein circulation takes place in the lymph vessels.

Protein circulation therefore requires a well-functioning lymph vessel system, otherwise the connective tissue becomes congested with

9 The lymph vessel system

the lymph-obligatory load. If protein remains in connective tissue for too long, its molecular structure changes and it is perceived by the body as foreign. The body will now activate its defensive system and break down the foreign protein. In addition, protein molecules attract water and thus promote oedema formation.

10 Equilibrium and balance as a goal of massage

10.1 Bathtub

In order to explain the problem "cosmetic or physiotherapeutic treatment with or without lymph drainage" again from another point of view, we draw a bathtub, the contents of which represent connective tissue. The inflow is filtration through the arterial system, the outflow resorption into the venous system. Every bathtub has an overflow drain to prevent flooding (this is the lymph vessel system) if we forget to turn off the taps. This should act as a safety valve. We have balanced conditions when the bathtub is full and inflow equals outflow. Starling has already described this 100 years ago. If the drain is blocked, that is resorption is not functioning properly, the water level climbs up to the overflow, which must now remove the excess water. The same is valid for the situation in which filtration outweighs resorption. The overflow drain of the bathtub, corresponding to the lymph vessel system, has a safety valve function. If for some reason this function is not fulfilled, oedema develops. The lymph vessel system is then no longer able to relieve the loose connective tissues of its load. This can be a water load, fat load, cell load or protein load. If the capacity of the overflow drain is exceeded or the drain is blocked for some reason, the bathtub will overflow. This condition then takes the form of oedema.

In practice this means that it always depends on the type of tissue whether and how we should combine circulation-stimulating methods with MLD.

If disturbances of the venous and/or lymph vessel system are present, the logical consequence is that the return-flow system is impaired and congestion – and possibly even an oedema – may develop in the connective tissue. If in a disturbed drainage situation such as this, filtration is increased by means of circulation-stimulating measures, this would be a grave error which would only serve to worsen the supply and drainage situation in the connective tissue, because increased circulation not only brings nutrients and oxygen into the tissue, which of course is very important, but also more water. Preventing this takes priority. Thus no circulation stimulation treatment in cases of impaired venous and lymph drainage!

10 Equilibrium and balance as a goal of massage

If our fingers feel soft, weak, spongy, waterlogged tissue, we would treat it with a few or no circulation-stimulating measures (massage, fangotherapy, hot air, irradiation, galvanization, hot or cold compresses, circulation masks) but rather with soothing and drainage promoting methods (Dr. Vodder's MLD). We would otherwise upset the fluid equilibrium.

If we feel firm, taut tissue, the entire range of circulation-stimulating methods may be applied, plus a short equalizing MLD.

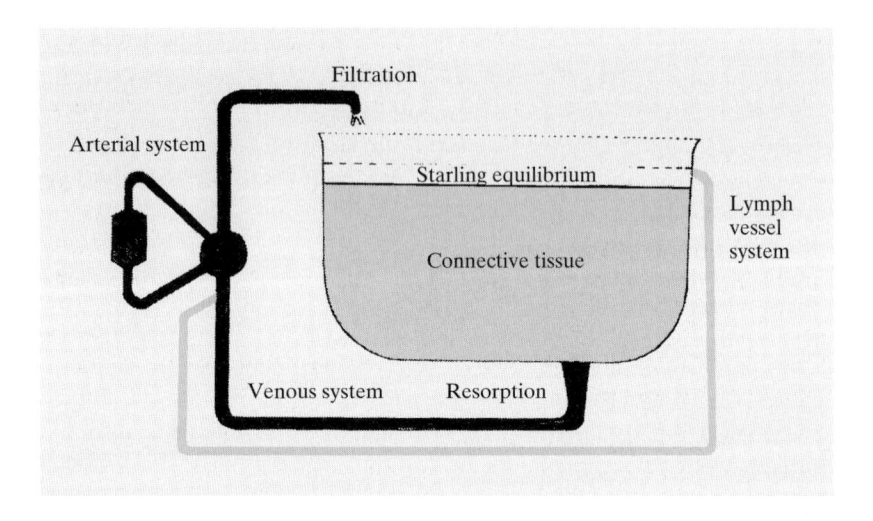

Fig. 9

If the bathtub has already overflowed, i.e. oedema has already developed, then under no circumstances should treatment be used that increases the load which must be transported by the lymph vessel system.

10.2 Fluid equilibrium

All circulation-promoting methods increase filtration into the tissue. In order to guarantee fluid equilibrium in the connective tissue it is always necessary, for safety reasons, to perform MLD. The intensity of the drainage depends on whether there are drainage problems in the tissue concerned. This is easy to determine by touch. Soft loose tissue is more likely to become oedematous and must be treated longer with MLD.

Circulation should then be stimulated carefully and in moderation. Firm, taut tissue can withstand more blood and requires less MLD. In the future MLD should be incorporated in cosmetic treatment and physiotherapy with these aspects in mind. Stimulate circulation first and conclude with MLD to maintain the fluid equilibrium.

10.3 Equilibrium in natural healing methods

All natural healing methods strive to produce a state of equilibrium in the organism. Consider the Chinese art of healing, acupuncture. An acupuncturist inserts needles in specific places along energy paths (meridians) in order to supply or remove energy and thus create balance in the energy paths.

Yoga derives from the Indian culture. It involves physical and spiritual training as well as movements containing elements of tension and relaxation with the goal of creating a balanced being. Therapists speak of equilibrium of the autonomic nervous system which maintains human health.

There is yin and yang, acid-alkaline balance, and many other examples in nature in which innate balanced interactions can be seen.

If we employ a circulation-stimulating measure, then drainage is the appropriate counterpart to guarantee fluid balance in the tissues i.e. MLD.

11 Oedema forms

In 1892, Winiwarter gave an excellent description of the development of lymphoedema:

"At first the skin does not look different, only a little taut. Pressing with a finger still causes a depression that remains, but the consistency of the skin and the subcutaneous tissue is more elastic and soft than doughy (as in the case of a simple oedema). When attempting to lift a fold of the tegument, one notices that the skin is thicker, more resistant, more tightly fixed to its foundation than is normal. Later, the consistency becomes progressively harder and more firm or only part of the extremity remains oedematous while the rest hardens. Gradually, after 5–10 years, the circumference of the limb reaches absolutely monstrous proportions due to swelling. Usually the lower leg has become a shapeless, uniformly thick cylinder similar to wide trousers gathered about the ankle and suddenly narrowing, or may have thick bulges and pendulous lobes in front hanging down to the instep or on the side hanging down to the ground like the folds of a gown while the foot itself has preserved normal dimension. If however, the elephantiasis has spread downward, the foot appears as a massive, formless lump ..."

The classical division of lymphoedema stems from Földi [18]. He separates oedema into three categories:

1. Lymphostatic oedema (due to mechanical insufficiency which is brought on by organic or functional changes).
2. Dynamic oedema (due to a dynamic insufficiency).
3. Safety-valve insufficiency of lymph drainage.

Oedema develops when the transport capacity of the lymph vessel system is not sufficient to transport the lymph-obligatory load out of the tissue. The lymph-obligatory load can vary according to the body region and the disease. Thus we distinguish between water load, fat load, protein load and cell load.

The lymph-time volume is the amount of lymph that is transported in a given unit of time.

If the lymph-obligatory load increases for some reason, oedema need not necessarily develop. The lymph-time volume increases, and thus also the frequency and amplitude of the lymph angion pulsations. Only if the lymph-time volume exceeds the transport capacity of the lymph vessel system will develop oedema.

As long as the increasing lymph-obligatory load is compensated, no oedema develops. This is a phase of *oedema susceptibility*. The body has its own methods for dealing with the risk of oedema:

- Neighboring lymph pathways increase their transport capacity and take on lymph from the damaged area.
- The body forms connections between lymph vessels, known as lymphatic anastomoses. Sometimes, there are also lymphovenous anastomoses.
- Prelymphatic pathways, which can be found in the adventitia of the large blood vessels, take up the prelymph and carry it to functioning lymph vessels.
- In a region at risk of oedema, monocytes from the blood migrate into the connective tissue, where they turn into macrophages. They then *break up* the proteins they find in the connective tissue, which is also known as proteolytic protein breakdown.

In this way the protein load is diminished. Thus the oedema develops if the extralymphatic cellular protein regulation fails and the lymph-time-volume exceeds the transport capacity for the lymph vessel system.

11.1 Lymphostatic oedema (protein-rich)

Lymphostatic oedema is oedema resulting from mechanical inadequacy of lymph drainage. This mechanical insufficiency can be **organic or functional** in origin.

Organic changes have to do with connective tissue and the prelymphatic paths within it; they also concern lymph vessels with developmental disorders. Lymph paths may be obstructed by tumors, inflammation, or (in Africa) by parasites. They may be damaged by cuts, operations, accidents, or x-rays. They can be constricted by tight clothing. There may be a paucity of lymph vessels.

Functional changes are temporary and may have to do with lymph vessels, i.e. if the valves do not close, the walls of the vessel are permeable, the motoricity of the lymph angions is disturbed, or contractions of the skeletal muscle are absent (e.g. paralytic stroke or insufficient movement). The vessels may be cramped or paralysed.

11 Oedema forms

Lymphostatic oedemas are further classified as primary and secondary. Primary oedemas are congenital (hereditory or sporadic). Secondary oedemas are those caused by a known disease.

The category of lymphostatic oedema has been extended by one type, first described by Price in 1970 [19]: endemic elephantiasis. It occurs in Ethiopia and results from walking around barefoot. Silicate and aluminium are absorbed through the skin, enter the lymphatic system and cause damage there. The result is oedema and elephantiasis. The fact that a term has been coined for this disease, *Lymphangioconosiss*, demonstrates the attempt to distinguish between the reaction of the lymphatic system to absorbed, inanimate particulate substances and typical lymphangitis.

11.2 Dynamic oedema (low-protein)

In dynamic insufficiency there is a normal, functional lymph vessel apparatus. As a result of excess fluid however, the lymph vessels can no longer remove the fluid from tissue. The result is a low-protein dynamic oedema.

It is only advantageous to apply Manual Lymph Drainage to oedema caused by mechanical insufficiency. Low-protein oedema is not affected by MLD because the forces causing the oedema are much stronger than the influence of the massage.

A kidney oedema is an example of a low-protein oedema, i.e. the kidney eliminates protein, which reduces the level of proteins in the blood. The colloid-osmotic pressure of the blood (oncotic suction of the blood proteins) is thus diminished. The capillary filters as usual but resorbs less. The result is a low-protein dynamic oedema.

The same holds true for hunger oedema. The colloid-osmotic pressure of the blood is also diminished, in this case due to the absence of dietary proteins. Thus the oncotic pressure of blood proteins sinks and a low-protein dynamic oedema results. It would be pointless to apply MLD to either of these oedema forms. It would not cause any damage but would not have a positive effect either.

Another type of low protein oedemas are those caused by heart insufficiency – the so called *heart oedemas* (congestive heart failure). Földi writes: 'The cardiac oedema is the result of a very complex process with

Dynamic oedema (low-protein) 11.2

a series of neural, hormonal, circulatory and renal disturbances. The heart musculature is weakened, leading to congestion in the right chamber of the heart and on into the venous system.' The increased pressure in the venous system extends to the capillaries, which Földi terms active hyperaemia. The result is increased filtration. The fluid volume cannot be processed by a normally-functioning lymph system. Therefore, the lymph vessels labor to a certain extent under a double load, since the inflow of the lymph of the thoracic duct is severely hindered by the sharply elevated pressure in the venous arch.

The lymph-obligatory water load exceeds the transport capacity of the lymph vessels. The disturbance can no longer be compensated, leading to haemodynamic insufficiency with a lymphostatic component due to congestion in the lymph vessels. This cardiac oedema is an absolute contraindication for Manual Lymph Drainage. Were we to perform MLD in this situation, we could possibly pump fluids into the heart via the lymphatic and venous systems, which could result in a pulmonary oedema.

Also enteropathic protein loss belongs to this category. Proteins are expelled with the stools. Ulceration of the intestinal mucous membrane leads to the escape of the lymph into the intestinal lumen. Likewise, a congenital abnormality could be the cause.

Varicose veins present a situation similar to heart oedema. An elevated intravascular pressure also exists in the veins, distal venules, and capillaries and due to dilation a column of blood – usually interrupted by valves – causes an elevated hydrostatic pressure. We therefore again have increased filtration with normal resorption. However the flow of lymph-obligatory load into the venous arch is not disturbed.

Some legs with varicose veins are also slender. The lymph vessel system functions efficiently and is capable of maintaining the Starling equilibrium. However there are legs with varicose veins that are oedematous. Both the venous system and the lymph vessel system are dysfunctional in this case.

Some legs with varicose veins are slender in the morning and thick in the evening. The lymph vessels are able to remove excess fluid from tissue for a while, but after a certain point the amount of filtrate exceeds the capacity transport of the lymph vessels and a low-protein dynamic oedema results. This type of oedema, created by an elevated hydrostatic venous pressure, cannot be cured with MLD. We do, however, treat varicose veins in order to stimulate the lymph vessels to perform optimally, i.e. do everything possible to stimulate the lymph vessel system. For this, other therapies are combined.

11.3 Safety-valve insufficiency

This is described by a sudden increase in the lymph-obligatory load and a total lymph congestion. If both disturbances occur simultaneously then a quantitative change is seen in the oedema as well as a qualitative change to the point of necrosis.

12 Cosmetic indications

- The first indication is the prevention of imbalance in the fluid equilibrium. Drainage is indicated after any circulation stimulating measure and should therefore be part of every cosmetic treatment.
- General regeneration is a very important indication. It is advisable to give 18 whole-body lymph drainage treatments at regular intervals (for explanation see "Connective-tissue").
- Acne is a major indication. To ensure success, frequent and long treatments should be given at the beginning of a series of treatments. The treatment time should be at least 30 minutes per session. At this stage we should warn you that a slight worsening of the acne might occur. For details we refer you to our courses.
- All congestive conditions such as rosacea, facial erythrosis, telangiectasis, facial oedema, and haematomas, the latter two also after face-lifting.
- Tear sacs, if they involve proteinaceous oedema.
- All skin alterations resulting from protein accumulation in the connective tissue or chronic injury: allergies, chronic eczema, burns, chronic inflammation (take precautions).
- Enhancement of general resistance.
- Scars become smaller, softer, and less visible.
- Favourable results have also been obtained in the treatment of old and new keloids.
- Panniculosis (*cellulite*) is a very important indication. Whether treatment can be combined in this case with circulatory stimulation depends on the drainage situation. Soft, spongy, waterlogged tissue will not tolerate circulatory stimulation of any kind.
- In maternal care, prevention of leg oedema by regular MLD and prevention of striae gavidarum (stretch marks) by timely skin care with MLD [20]. With much treatment, pre-existing stretch marks can improve with MLD. A skin alteration caused by lymph blockage (lymphostatic skin alterations) can lead to the disorder *cutis striate lymphostatica*. The histological picture reveals damage to the elastic and collagen fibres. We may therefore assume that prophy-

12 Cosmetic indications

lactic MLD will prevent the appearance of this disorder or restrict the alterations to mild forms.

- Thick legs, heavy legs, fatigued legs.
- Fasting cures combined with MLD will maintain skin tautness.
- Mastodynia: this is described as the tension women feel in their breasts after ovulation, which can develop into pain. This tension pain can also be traced back to lymph congestion, among other things. Regular MLD can provide relief here.

13 Indications for physiotherapy

The reader is referred to the "Compendium" of Dr. Vodder's Manual Lymph Drainage by Dr. Kasseroller, the medical director of the Vodder School.

Finally, there are the abstracts of the Society of Dr. Vodder's Manual Lymph Drainage [Gesellschaft für Manuelle Lymphdrainage nach Dr. Vodder], where the lectures given at the society's continuing education seminars are published.

14 Relative contraindications (precautions)

- MLD can be used in cases of thyroid hyperactivity, but the area of the thyroid itself should be avoided. Do not treat profundus-terminus, but rather occiput-terminus. In general, decrease the treatment periods somewhat. MLD must feel pleasant to receive.
- Asthmatic bronchial attacks are triggered by the vagus nerve. Since MLD also has an effect on the vagus nerve, there is a danger that MLD may precipitate an attack. For this reason begin treatment of asthmatic patients in the attack-free period. The treatment times should not be longer than 45 minutes. Omit the manipulation on the sternum.
- Lymph nodes which were once affected by tuberculosis are also contraindicated. There is a danger that encapsulated bacilli may again be activated by the massage.
- If a nevus represents a precancerous state, omit this area from MLD treatment.
- Do not perform abdominal treatment during menstruation.
- Low blood pressure: In such cases a whole-body treatment should never be performed at the beginning, as this would only depress the blood pressure even further. It is best to begin with a small area and increase it in the course of time. It has been observed that blood pressure stabilizes as a result.
- Treatment of chronic inflammation must begin with short treatment sessions that emphasize diversity.
- Treated cancer: lymphoedema is often an unfortunate consequence of cancer treatment. This lymphoedema is an indication for Manual Lymph Drainage, albeit **only** for properly-trained therapists.

In the above conditions MLD can be carried out, but only in combination with special precautions.

Under no circumstances should estheticians attempt to treat a client's illness.

Treatment should be terminated whenever an effect is felt to be unpleasant. The general rule applies: Dr. Vodder's Lymph Drainage must always be experienced as pleasant.

15 Absolute contraindications

The absolute contraindications are:

- All malignant diseases and
- all acute inflammations with infection, as well as
- acute allergic reactions.

The reason is the same in all cases: degenerate cells, bacteria, viruses and allergens are transported by the lymph vessel system. If MLD were used, these could be forced through the nodes where they would normally be attacked and broken down. Ultimately they would find their way into the blood and spread through the whole body. This would be a disaster.

- Because of the associated risk of embolism, recent thrombosis is also contraindicated.
- The so-called heart oedema (congestive heart failure) arising from insufficiency of the right side of the heart is an absolute contraindication (see dynamic oedema).

16 Treatment guidelines

16.1 Excursus in the cosmetic field

Let us examine what services estheticians perform for their customers and what effects they have.

They massage, apply compresses – hot or cold, do vapozones, perform peelings, carry out electrical stimulation therapy, perform iontophoresis, prepare circulation masks, and apply thermal masks. All these measures stimulate the circulation.

The majority of the treatments applied at a beauty institute are related to stimulate blood circulation – from a physiological point of view an extremely one-sided treatment. Circulation, of course, is essential for supplying nutrients and oxygen to the tissue, but water also enters the tissue. Increased blood circulation opens the capillaries, and filtering is thus increased. MLD would counter this effect by transporting excess fluid out of the tissues. A good approach is: first stimulation of blood flow and then manual lymph drainage. In this way nutrients are offered and supplied quickly to the cells because transit distance and thus diffusion time are short.

Examples of treatment guidelines:

16.2 Inflammations

Since inflammation, in addition to various types of oedema, is one of the main indications, we should discuss which forms of inflammation are indicated and which contraindicated.

Inflammation has five distinguishing features: **redness**, resulting from increased circulation, **swelling**, which results from enhanced permeability of the capillary walls and increased exudation, as does the sensation of **heat**. The release of histamine from mast cells causes **pain**. Also, there is **functional impairment** of the inflamed area.

Inflammations always take the same course. They are the body's response to an irritation or damage. It doesn't matter whether it's a wound, burn, bacterial infection or allergens. Depending on the tissue's reaction, either the inflammation heals or scar tissue is formed, or it becomes chronic, or even leads to histolysis. Inflammation occurs in the

Inflammations 16.2

loose connective tissue. The following is an abbreviated description of the course of an inflammation. The first manifestation is histamine production, which shifts the pH of the ground substance into the acid region. The arterioles open up and the capillaries become distended. Vessel walls become more permeable, pain receptors are sensitized. Blood becomes more viscous, leading finally to stasis. Swelling results. Leukocytes drift into this changed tissue and attempt to phagocytose the pathogen. Necrotic tissue is also phagocytosed. The phagocytes die and, along with the liquefied ground substance, are excreted as pus or broken down by macrophages. Now lymphocytes drift into this region and switch off the inflammation-triggering antigens. Finally, the antigen-antibody complexes are eliminated by eosinophilic granulocytes; the inflammation is now healed. Not all inflammations proceed through all of these phases. It is entirely possible for incoming leukocytes to cause the inflammation to subside right at the beginning. If the antigens are not fully decomposed, or if the acute phase proceeds weakly, then disruptive factors can be left behind, leading to a chronic inflammation.

The lymph vessels react differently from the blood capillaries: in the inflamed centre they dilate so that the lymphangion valves no longer close. The lymph vessels proximal to the inflammation, close spastically. This reaction can be life-saving in cases where the inflammation is caused by toxic substances. These substances are bound to protein and must be transported through the lymph system. They would ultimately lead to blood poisoning if this mechanism did not arrest the inflammation-producing substances until the phagocytosis system has a chance to consume them and break them down. Thus, in the case of acute inflammation caused by poisons, bacteria, viruses or allergens, MLD is contraindicated. Under the influence of MLD, the toxins could be pushed through the lymph before being eliminated by our immune system. They would then find their way into the blood stream, causing blood poisoning. In cases where inflammation is not caused by toxins, bacteria or viruses, MLD is the therapy of choice. Examples are cases due to irritation like epicondylitis or chronic inflammations, in which the inflammatory substances have been largely broken down. The therapist must therefore always consider whether MLD will spread or reduce inflammation on the basis of the above points.

If the loose connective tissue is restored to a normal state through MLD therapy, the inflammation is healed, i.e. all pathogens have been transported out of the connective tissue. In the normalised connective tissue the capillary filtrate is also restored to normal. The acidic milieu is neutralized.

16.3 Acne

Acne in its various forms constitutes a serious problem for the esthetician. The causes are so numerous that we cannot simply say: first eliminate the causes and then treat the symptoms. That would require specialists from various medical fields.

From our point of view acne is an accumulation of inflamed hair follicles due to the conversion of sebum into fatty acid under the influence of the bacteria Corynum and Staphylococcus albus. The signs of inflammation are redness, swelling, pain and heat. Nearly all forms of acne manifest these symptoms. Excellent results are obtained by treating acne by means of MLD, provided that certain principles are observed. At first the acne must be treated with 30-minute therapy sessions every day: in the first week at least five times, the second week – at least three times, the third week at least twice, etc. Before treatment a circulation mask should be applied (do not clean each time). Do not wash the face with soap or alcohol. Use a hydrophilic oil, if possible three times a day. Good digestion and proper eating habits, perhaps involving a change in diet, should be a goal. Drink much fluids – water or herbal tea. If these principles are observed, it shouldn't be difficult to eliminate the acne. It is then only a question of time. Acne must be treated intensively and over a long period if favorable results are to be obtained. As mentioned earlier, sometimes acne appears worse after the first treatment.

If the acne to be treated is on the chest or back, we apply a hot compression of horsetail infusion for 10 minutes followed by MLD for 30 minutes with outstanding results.

16.4 Cellulite (panniculopathia – oedemato – fibrosclerotica) [46]/Adiposis

Cellulite is commonly described as the appearance of an indented or orange peel skin. One should always differentiate between adiposis and panniculopathia-oedemato-fibrosclerotica (the so-called cellulite). In women, there is often an accumulation of fat cells in the abdomen and outer sides of the thighs. This is a characteristic of the female body. The view of this as beautiful or not has changed substantially. If we look at the paintings of Rubens for example, all of his female characters are shown with a massive cellulite. Whether these are adipose figures or if these women really suffered from the so called cellulite cannot be seen in these representations. MLD can be used successfully with adiposis. However other methods must also be used, especially diet reduction. Vitamins are very important as they are needed for metabolism of stored fat. Nutrient intake must be reduced so that the body breaks down the fat depots and converts them to energy. Gymnastics can be done to tone the affected tissues. A daily cleansing with hydrophilic oil has proven helpful and has a similar effect to the Kneipp hydrotherapy treatments.

Whether MLD can be combined with circulatory stimulating methods depends on the feel of the tissues. If it feels soft and spongy, stimulation would be inappropriate because only more water would be pumped into an already congested tissue, obviously suffering from drainage problems. If the tissue feels firm we are dealing with solid fat and circulatory stimulation followed by MLD can be used without a second thought. There need not be any fear that the skin will become flabby after weight loss because we specifically treat these areas. On the contrary, the tone of the tissues increases with MLD.

Therefore, so-called *cellulite* or medically speaking *panniculopathia-oedemato-fibrosclerotica* is, according to Curri [46], a pathological condition of the fat tissue. With *cellulite*, one shouldn't speak of fat accumulation, rather a structural disturbance of the fat tissue. The fat content is normal in *cellulite*. The local increase in volume can be traced back to the formation of micro and macro nodules, small and large nodes. Besides this, fibres multiply and surround the fat cells. Please note that *cellulite* is a disease of the fat tissue. This can occur in overweight, normal or thin people. Also *cellulite* is always related to venous congestion and in many cases to lymph congestion.

In the first stages of *cellulite* there is not yet a venous insufficiency but an increased capillary permeability. This isn't primarily caused by damage to the endothelium, rather by a disturbance of the pericapillary tissue, i.e. the connective tissue and its components. An oedema thus slowly develops in the interstitium of the fat tissue which pushes apart the fat cells. How does the fat tissue react now to this flooding? Some of

16 Treatment guidelines

the fat cells are destroyed so that fat mixes with the surrounding fluid. Each fat cell is wrapped by reticular fibres which thicken and multiply forming a type of capsule. These fibres transform into collagen fibres and result in a sclerotic connective tissue during the course of the "Cellulite". This is nodule formation. If more of these nodules combine and become surrounded by a thick connective tissue capsule, they can be felt as nodes. This already represents the final stage of the process.

Curri distinguishes 4 stages of *cellulite*:

1. Flooding of the interstitium.
2. Increased puffiness, i.e. the tissue becomes softer.
3. Many small nodules and some large nodes (macronodules). An examination technique at this point is to take a fold of skin firmly and hold it for 3–4 seconds. Upon release the patient experiences pain.
4. In the fourth stage, the so called orange peel skin develops, nodes can be felt and there is pain.

It should be noted that these four stages do not develop evenly. It is entirely possible that all stages occur at the same time. These circumstances enable us to say that we can achieve very good results with cellulite using Manual Lymph Drainage. According to Curri, the third and fourth stages of *cellulite* are the final stages and cannot be altered by any therapy. However because all stages are found at the same time, it is always correct to apply MLD. Also, this condition begins with an inundation of the interstitium, i.e. it is always associated with an oedema. *Cellulite* is never an inflammation. In many different ways the relationship between the smallest vessels and the tissue are disrupted. Think of venous congestion and also the effect of the birth control pill. The effect of female hormones on the ground substance of connective tissue is known. Oestrogen polymerizes the hyaluronic acid of the ground substance; progesterone or testosterone depolymerise and disrupt the chain structure of hyaluronic acid. During the menstrual cycle one can imagine a type of balance occurring which would be severely disturbed by the pill. Curri [46] has shown in experiments that MLD combined with a simultaneous application of the cream Celuvase, brings about a significant improvement. It is a question of an effective treatment method absolutely free of side effects.

16.5 Lipoedema

Now a word about lipoedema. Here we have a symmetrical saddle-like storage of fat especially on the buttocks and the legs but also on the arms. The feet and hands are normal (oedema free). There is a free transition between lipoedema and cellulite. After a certain time cellulite can also develop. Nodes are often visible and palpable in lipoedema. Lipoedema is a very good indication for MLD. Many patients suffering from lipoedema complain of pain especially during over exertion of the legs. Bandaging of the legs should be a necessity but is often not possible due to the pain or inability to wear them – at least until after a few MLD treatments. Lipoedema can be aggravated by venous insufficiency or an initial lymphatic component.

There is a big difference between an adiposis, which is a general storage of fat and a localised lipoedema. Even a diet would not help a Lipoedema patient to lose weight and decrease oedematous areas. Yet any increase of weight must be avoided. The underpinning scientific theories have shown us how to treat these patients: Dr. Vodder's Manual Lymph Drainage ranks highly as a basic treatment. In addition we combine compression bandages and hydrotherapy in appropriate cases.

16.6 Toothaches

Under certain circumstances MLD can evoke pain in the teeth and jaws – namely, if the patient has a focus in the dental region. Dead teeth can give rise to granulomas that are activated by MLD and become painful. If a festering tooth is extracted and appropriate care not received, residual ostitis may form which also reacts to MLD. On the other hand, toothaches can also be eliminated using MLD, depending on their cause.

16.7 Consideration of outside temperature

The therapist must take even the outside temperature into account when treating a patient because it has an effect on the skin capillaries.

Body temperature is regulated by the blood. In order to cope with extreme fluctuations in outside temperature (e.g. winter: $-20°$ C; summer:

+30° C) and still maintain a constant temperature, the body has regulatory mechanisms. In a cold environment the blood circulates as much as possible in the core of the body in order to reduce heat loss to the outside. When the outside temperature is high, the blood flows beneath the skin so that the capillaries dilate and heat is dissipated to the outside. The capillary dilation however results in a large quantity of filtrate. This must be taken into consideration during therapy. On hot days, circulatory-stimulating methods risk upsetting the Starling equilibrium. In summer, therefore, emphasis should be placed on drainage and MLD with less circulatory stimulation and vice-versa in winter.

16.8 Iontophoresis

If iontophoresis and MLD are combined to introduce active agents into the body, certain factors should be considered. It is not very advantageous to perform MLD after iontopheresis, because the substances introduced into the tissues are eventually removed again by drainage. On the other hand, galvanic current used in iontophoresis dilates the capillaries so that the blood flow is increased, resulting in more filtrate in the connective tissue. MLD should therefore be carried out after iontophoresis, in order to maintain the Starling equilibrium. So as not to impair the effect of iontophoresis, it should **not be combined with** MLD. For clients that are oedematous or show a tendency to become so, iontophoresis would be inappropriate. Palpating will again reveal the state of the tissue. Soft, spongy connective tissue is in any case more oedema-prone than taut tissue. Iontophoresis on oedema-prone patients, as is often performed on cellulite, always presents special problems.

16.9 Stress and Dr. Vodder's Manual Lymph Drainage

Now I would like to say something about **stress** [33]. Basically stress is a useful, life-saving alarm reaction which enables us to react immediately with a flight or fight response.

In the *civilised* world, stress has degenerated because we are exposed to it day-in and day-out and can't escape from it. Because of this, severe injury and illness can occur as we cannot go through the so called *stress mechanism*. In the moment of the stress situation the brain waves abruptly change. This has a direct effect on the autonomic nervous system, via the hypothalamus. The sympathetic response puts the body into an alarm state which means: increased blood pressure and pulse, release of the flight hormone adrenalin and the aggression hormone noradrenalin. Fat and carbohydrate reserves are mobilised. The result is a decrease in the skin resistance, caused by an increased sweat secretion through anxiety. The normal reaction to stress is the transition to movement, i.e. flight, fight or another energy deployment such as shrieking. This brings about a normal autonomic state.

Modern stress, which has a continual weakening effect on us, has no outlet because a series of restrictions imposed by civilization prevent this instinctive impulse. The result is damage to the circulation, digestive tract and immune system. Muscles, joints and lungs are damaged by deposits and an accelerated aging process. At the same time, sensitivity to other stress factors is increased. When the nutrients are unused, the fatty acids convert to cholesterol and are deposited on the vessel walls. The result is arteriosclerosis. Through a shift in the hormonal balance the autonomic system is disturbed, e.g. increased strain on the circulation and risk of infarction. Hydrochloric acid production in the stomach is stimulated and the intestines tend to cramp. Even the structure of the collagen in the connective tissue changes.

Now since Manual Lymph Drainage has a sympathicolytic effect, it is in a position to break down the stress reaction and thus helps to prevent stress from making us ill.

This only concerns the effect of MLD on the nervous system. By draining the tissue and removing wastes from the loose connective tissue, I believe that hormones activated by the stress reaction are taken away. A familiar quote of Vodder's was: "lymph drainage normalizes".

When talking of connective tissue one should also think of the connective tissue in the vessel walls. Manual Lymph Drainage works here in the same way. Looking at it this way, MLD is a rehabilitation method of the first degree.

The most severe lymphoclasia occur in the lymph nodes and other lymphatic organs, especially in acute strain as in stressful situations. Lymphoclasia in general refers to the breakdown of lymphocytes by macrophages of the reticuloendothelial or histiocytic system. Clasma(cy)tosis describes the process of phagocytosis of aged and/or damaged lymphocytes by clasmatocytes (histiocytes). In the germinal centres of the lymph nodes and spleen, both lymphopoiesis (lymphocyte formation) and lymphoclasia (lymphocyte breakdown) occur.

16.10 Scars

Scars are formed from connective tissue. Often the repair reaction is excessive, resulting in the formation of keloids. These keloids are raised above the normal skin level. They contain more water and soluble collagen than normal scars. Both formation of scar tissue can be reduced or even prevented by the regular application of MLD. Even the reddish discolouration of the scar disappears under the influence of MLD. Oedema forms along fresh laceration scars and around the edge of large-surface burn scars. It is important to drain this area. The objective of the treatment is to render the scar stable and elastic, prevent shrinkage, revascularise the tissue, reduce discolouration and itching, reduce the scar to the normal skin level, eliminate fibrosis and normalise the tissue surrounding the scar, i.e. in most cases reduce oedema. Normally scar tissue is treated with MLD like the skin lymph drainage. Exceptions are made in the treatment of secondary lymphoedema following cancer operations or after 3rd degree burns. Hutzschenreuter determined experimentally that revascularisation proceeds significantly more rapidly when scars are treated with Manual Lymph Drainage. Full-body treatment at regular intervals is recommended for large-scale scars: in this manner, we influence the organ connective tissue, which has a favorable effect on scar-tissue regeneration.

An observation made in Central America is worth noting: in dark-skinned people scars are white, which, of course, is very conspicuous. When these scars are treated with MLD, a pigmentation process takes place [42] and the scar takes on the normal skin colour.

Part II
Practical Section

1 Massage technique

Dr. Vodder's Manual Lymph Drainage can be included in the classical large-surface massage methods. To some extent, the manual techniques even resemble the large, decongestive manipulation of classical massage. A close examination, however, will reveal that MLD is considerably more difficult as it involves manual techniques that are not used in any classical form of massage. All massage techniques have one thing in common: by contacting the skin they stimulate specific receptors, resulting in a specific reaction. Which type of receptors are stimulated with the corresponding effect depends on how the skin is touched. To achieve the effects of Dr. Vodder's Manual Lymph Drainage it is required that this method be applied in its original form, as taught at the Dr. Vodder School in Walchsee.

We distinguish between four different techniques:

1.1 Stationary circles

The fingers are placed flat on the skin and it is moved either in the same place as stationary circles or in continuous spirals. The manipulations are used primarily for treating the neck, face and lymph nodes. The stationary circles are varied on the body and extremities by making circles – 5 circles in one spot – hand-on-hand or with eight fingers placed next to each other. In the latter case the fingers turn together in the same direction to move the skin in circles or alternating. The direction of pressure is determined by the lymph drainage. The fingers lie flat, sometimes the whole hand. Each of these circles is performed with a smooth increase of pressure into the tissue and a smooth decrease of pressure.

1.2 Pump technique

With this technique the palms are face downward. The thumb and fingers move together in the same direction, moving the skin in oval circles. This movement of thumb and fingers is controlled by the exaggerated movements of the wrist. The fingers are outstretched; the fingertips have no function in this technique. The wrist moves like a hinge. The forward motion of the fingers is carried out with pressure (as the wrist drops), the forward motion of the wrist is without pressure.

1.3 Scoop technique

In contrast to the pump technique with the scoop technique the palm is facing upward. Vodder describes the movement as a giving motion. The rotating wrist creates a corkscrew movement of the wrist-hand unit. The fingers are outstretched and swing towards the body during the pressure phase. Pressure is on the inward part of the stroke with no pressure on the outward stroke. The pivot point is the metacarpal-carpal joint of the index finger, whereby all the metacarpo-phalangeal joints are in contact with the skin during the pressure phase.

1.4 Rotary technique

This technique is used on relatively flat areas of the body and consists of various individual movements. The wrist moves up and down. As it moves down it swings from the outside toward the inside. The whole palm lies on the skin and turns it on an inward spiral. The thumb also makes circular movements in the direction of the lymph drainage of the skin. These motions are performed during the pressure phase. In the pressureless phase the wrist is raised and the four outstretched fingers move on and the thumb slides inward. Wrist moves down, the whole hand touches the skin (pressureless) and it begins to reapply pressure.

MLD consists of these four techniques, which may be combined during treatment. It can be seen from the description that Dr. Vodder's MLD consists of a combination of round or oval, small or large, deep or shallow circular movements. The skin is moved rather than stroked. For the purpose of instruction, this principle is handled generously in basic courses so that the direction of the movements becomes second nature to the student.

Precise execution of the manual technique is then practiced in more advanced courses.

1.5 Frequency of massage

The length of treatment of a particular body part, the use of certain pressure and the speed of movements can be explained, but not taught. Thus, the theoretical lessons are only an aid to explain the effect of

MLD and prepare the ground for an understanding of the value and application of MLD in physical therapy and health care. The dosage of MLD however, must depend on the fingertip control and intuition of the therapist and cannot be taught because in practice no two cases are identical.

Berta Bobath described in 1984 the Bobath concept: "However much we have learned and changed and continue to do both, it must be emphasised that every basic concept has not changed. Each therapist works differently with her/his experiences and personality. This is positive and creative. However, we all base our treatment on the same concept. This concept is so far reaching and open that it enables us to expand our learning and follow the continual developments in scientific research as well as the changes in the symptoms of the disease". We want to fully apply this statement to Dr. Vodder's Manual Lymph Drainage. The description of MLD must be seen and understood from this perspective.

Since the effect of MLD is largely derived from a mechanical displacement of fluids and the substances they carry, it is essential that the manual techniques developed by Vodder be precisely executed. Experience shows that the more exact the technique is, the better the results are. The use of a particular pressure depends on the state of the tissue to be treated. One could say: the softer the tissue, the lighter the pressure.

1.6 Environmental conditions for optimal therapy

For an optimal treatment, certain environmental factors are taken into account. Then the full effect can be felt on the nervous system without external disturbances, as well as the mechanical effect:

1. Conversation during therapy diverts attention and prevents autonomic changes. The patient should concentrate on the feelings in the skin. The attunement of the autonomic system will then be evoked via the skin senses.
2. The same applies to interruptions in the treatment, e.g. if the telephone rings, a new patient arrives, noise is made or the patient's calm is disturbed in any other way.
3. The patient's table should be comfortable – not so soft that he or she sinks in, but under no circumstance too hard.

1 Massage technique

4. The room should not be too hot or too cold but comfortably warm to promote relaxation. The indifference temperature for heat and cold receptors in the skin is 33° C.
5. The patient should not be dazzled by the glare of lights.
6. The skin contact zones should neither be too smooth, rough or moist. It is recommended that 2–3 drops of oil be used in treating the individual parts of the body. This will equalise the moisture of the skin. Under no circumstances should so much oil be used that one glides over the skin, as is the case in classical massage.

1.7 Basic principles

The following are a number of basic principles that are characteristic of MLD.

1. The proximal area is treated before the distal so that the proximal area is emptied to make room for fluid flowing in from the distal region.
2. MLD prescribes a certain degree of pressure limited to 30–40 mm/Hg.
3. Each circular movement has a variance in pressure from about 0 to about 20–30–40 mm/Hg, depending on the palpatory findings. The pressure is changed smoothly so that a pumping action is produced in the tissue.
4. The direction of pressure depends on the efferent lymph vessels in the skin.
5. The techniques and variations are repeated rhythmically, usually 5 to 7 times, either at the same location in stationary circles or in continuous spirals. Less frequent repetition is pointless because the inertial mass of the tissue fluid needs some time before it responds.
6. The pressure phase of a circle lasts longer than the relaxation phase.
7. As a rule, no reddening of the skin should appear.
8. MLD should not elicit pain.
9. Circles are made **with** the skin and not **on** the skin.

1.8 Sequence of manipulations

I Treatment of the neck (patient supine)

1. All rotary motions of the hand or fingers are towards the little finger side.
2. Effleurage: Five fan-shaped strokes with the thumbs flat from the sternum to the axilla. The last stroke is along the clavicle (collarbone).
3. Drainage of cervical lymph nodes: Stationary circles over the lymph nodes at the profundus, middle, and terminus with five circles at each point. 3 x.
4. Occiput: Stationary circles beginning at the base of the skull, following the cervical vertebrae and finishing in the terminus. 3 x.
5. Stationary circles: three positions from the tip of the chin to the profundus then profundus, middle, and terminus. 3 x.
6. Fork technique: Stationary circles in front (parotid) and behind the ears then profundus, middle, and terminus. 3 x.
7. Shoulder: Stationary circles moving the shoulders: over the ball of the shoulder, two positions on the trapezius border then the terminus. 3 x.
8. Stationary circles moving the shoulder from the acromium along the clavicle (fingers flat on the skin above the acromioclavicular joint) up to the terminus. 3 x.
9. Stationary circles on the profundus, middle and terminus. 1 x.
10. Final effleurage. 1 x.

1 Massage technique

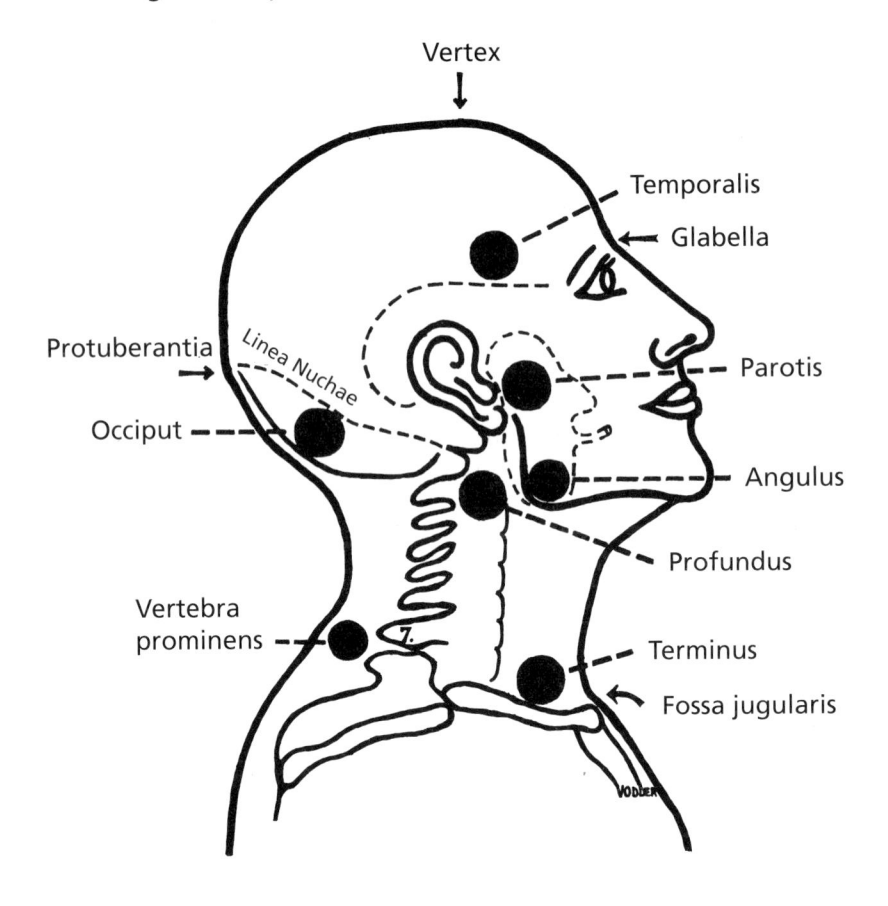

Fig. 10: Treatment points

II Treatment of the face (stand behind the patient's head)

1. Effleurage: parallel strokes below the lower lip, above the upper lip, nose, cheeks, and forehead.
2. Stationary circles starting at the midline below the lower lip, mid jaw then angle of the jaw, five circles at each point. 3 x.
3. Stationary circles from the midline above the upper lip, at the corners of the mouth then angle of the jaw. 3 x. Then profundus, middle, terminus, using the index finger in the terminus. 1 x.
4. Stationary circles from the bridge of the nose laterally to the cheek: from the tip of the nose 3 x, from the middle of the nose 3 x, from the root of the nose 3 x. Then down the sides of the nose from the root to the nostrils. 1 x.
5. The long journey: Stationary circles in three places: below the eyes with flat fingers, at the corners of the mouth and the tip of the chin; then spirals to the profundus (or stationary circles). 3 x.
6. Treatment of the eyes:
   - If necessary, the tear sacs should be treated now with stationary circles and half pressure (15 mm/Hg) using one or two fingers. 3 x.
   - Pull up several times with the index finger at the root of the nose. 3 x.
   - Press the eyebrows 5 times with the thumb and the flat index finger. 3 x.
   - With the thumbs at the root of the nose, pull up, rotate inward without pressure at the glabella and roll out over the eyebrows. 3 x.
7. Stationary circles with the fingers on the eyebrows, start with the index fingers (three places). 3 x.
8. Stationary circles with flat fingers from the middle of the forehead to the temples (three places). 3 x.
9. Stationary circles, two positions in front of the ears and profundus. 3 x.
10. Empty the profundus reservoir with 20 circles or more (always in sets of five).

1 Massage technique

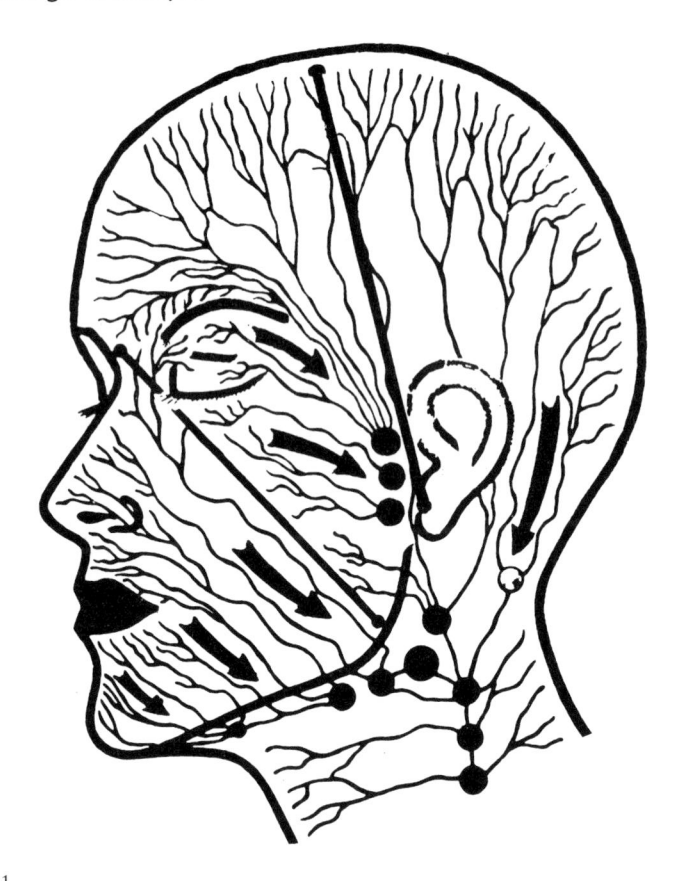

Fig. 11

11. Stationary circles over the profundus, middle and terminus. 1 x.

12. Effleurage:

- Stroke 3 times with the ball of the thumb (thenar eminence) from the glabella to the temples.
- Repeat the same movement to the temples, then turn the hand inward a quarter of a turn. Place the thumbs under the eyes and stroke lightly to the side across the cheeks. 3 x.
- Cup both hands carefully over the face. Relax and part the hands, stroking out to the sides. 3 x.
- Stroke laterally over the chin to the angle of the jaw. 3 x.

III Treatment of the arms

1. Long effleurage. 1 x.
2. Alternating scoop technique on the upper arm beginning with the inner hand. 3 x.
3. Pump technique over the deltoid muscle with one hand. 3 x.
4. Alternate circles with flat hands on each side of the deltoid muscle (hand washing motion). 3 x.
5. Stationary circles with 8 fingers on the upper arm lymph nodes, pressure towards the fingertips (direction of drainage towards the axilla). 3 x.
6. Pump – push alternating along the lateral side of the upper arm. 3 x.
7. Elbows: press with 4 fingers and the thumb. 3 x. Thumb circles around the lateral epicondyle in two lines. 3 x. Crease of the elbow with the thumb in a spiral motion, medial to lateral. Pressure goes medial. 3 x.
8. Scoop technique on forearm, supinated 3 x, then pronated 3 x, using the same hand to scoop.
9. Thumb circles alternating in three lines over the wrist. 3 lines, 3 x each.
10. Thumb circles alternating over the back of the hand beginning with the little finger side. 3 lines, 3 x each.
11. Thumb: with three thumb circles (index finger supports) then two pressings. 3 x.
12. Treat 2 fingers at a time making alternate circles with thumbs (index fingers support). Index and ring finger, middle and little finger. 3 x.
13. Palm of the hand with thumb circles alternating, 3 x, then parallel 3 x.
14. Final long effleurage. 1 x.

1 Massage technique

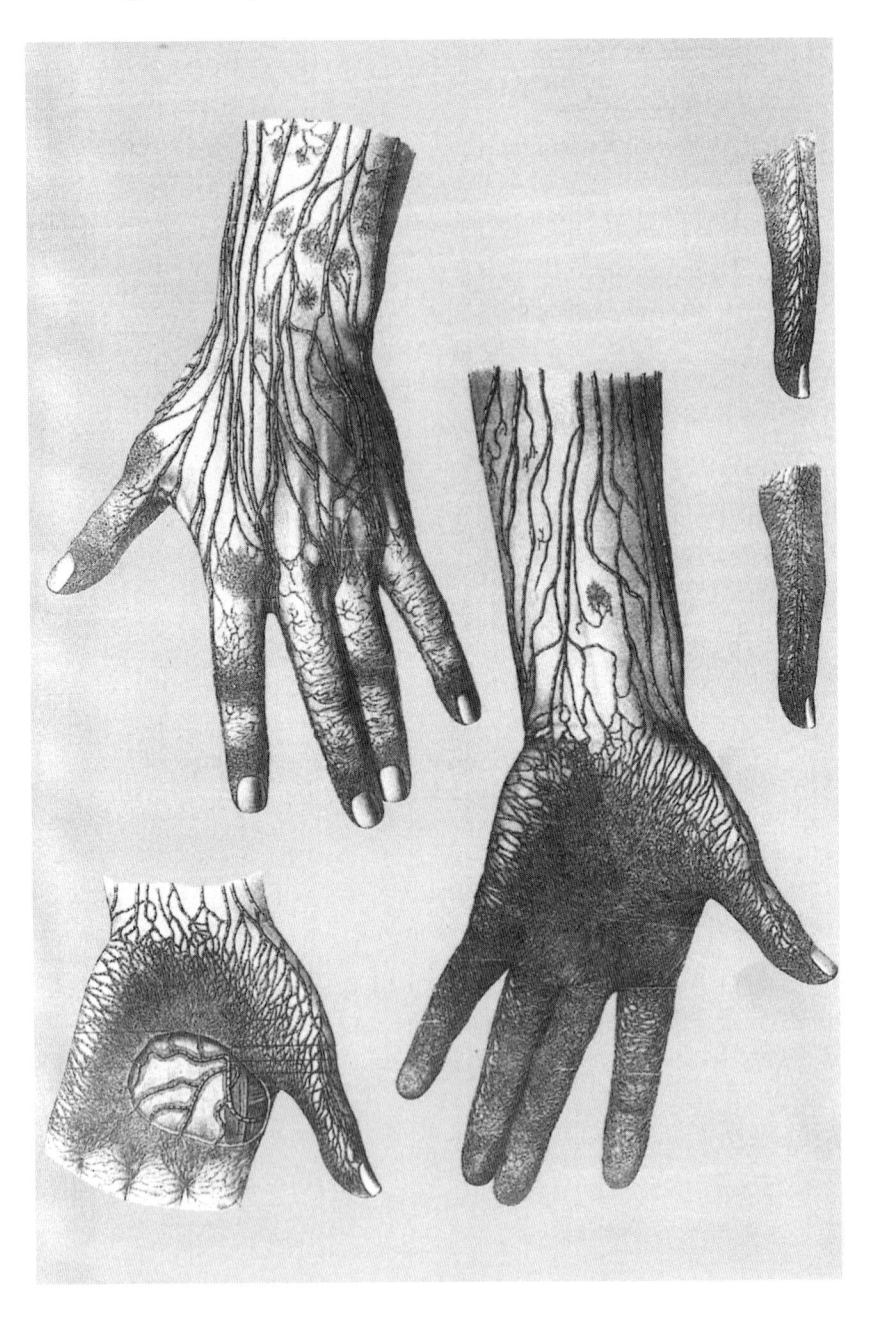

Fig. 12

IV Treatment of the legs

1. Long effleurage. 1 x.
2. Pump technique alternating on the anterior side of the thigh. 3 x.
3. Pump – push along on the medial, anterior, and lateral side of the thigh. 3 x each. On the medial side push with 4 fingers and on the anterior and lateral side push with the thumb.
4. Treat inguinal lymph nodes with stationary circles on 3 positions, using 8 fingers, flat and on a diagonal upwards. 3 x. Pressure is towards the fingertips (direction of drainage towards the inguinal lymph nodes) with circles toward the head. Then 3 continuous circles down to the knee with pressure on the upward part of the stroke. 1 x.
5. Treatment of the knee:
   - Pump – push along on the cauliflower. 3 x.
   - Scoop technique in the hollow of the knee with 8 flat fingers, distal to proximal. 3 x.
   - Patella (knee cap): leave the fingers in the hollow and now make thumb circles on each side of the patella. 3 x.
   - Pump technique with one hand over the knee. 3 x.
   - Treat the Pes anserinus with alternating thumb circles. 3 x.
6. Lower leg with the knee flexed:
   - Alternate between pump technique with one hand over the shin and scoop with the other hand over the calf. 3 x.
   - Alternating scoop technique with the thumbs running parallel to the shin bone. 3 x.
7. Extend leg again: parallel, 4-finger spirals on each side of the Achilles tendon. 3 x.
8. Ankle with alternating thumb circles. 3 lines, 3 x each.
9. Dorsum of the foot with thumb circles alternating. 3 lines, 3 x each.
10. Parallel thumb circles (oedema technique) on lymph sea. 3 x.
11. Pressing within the transverse arch. 3 x.
12. Final effleurage. 1 x.

1 Massage technique

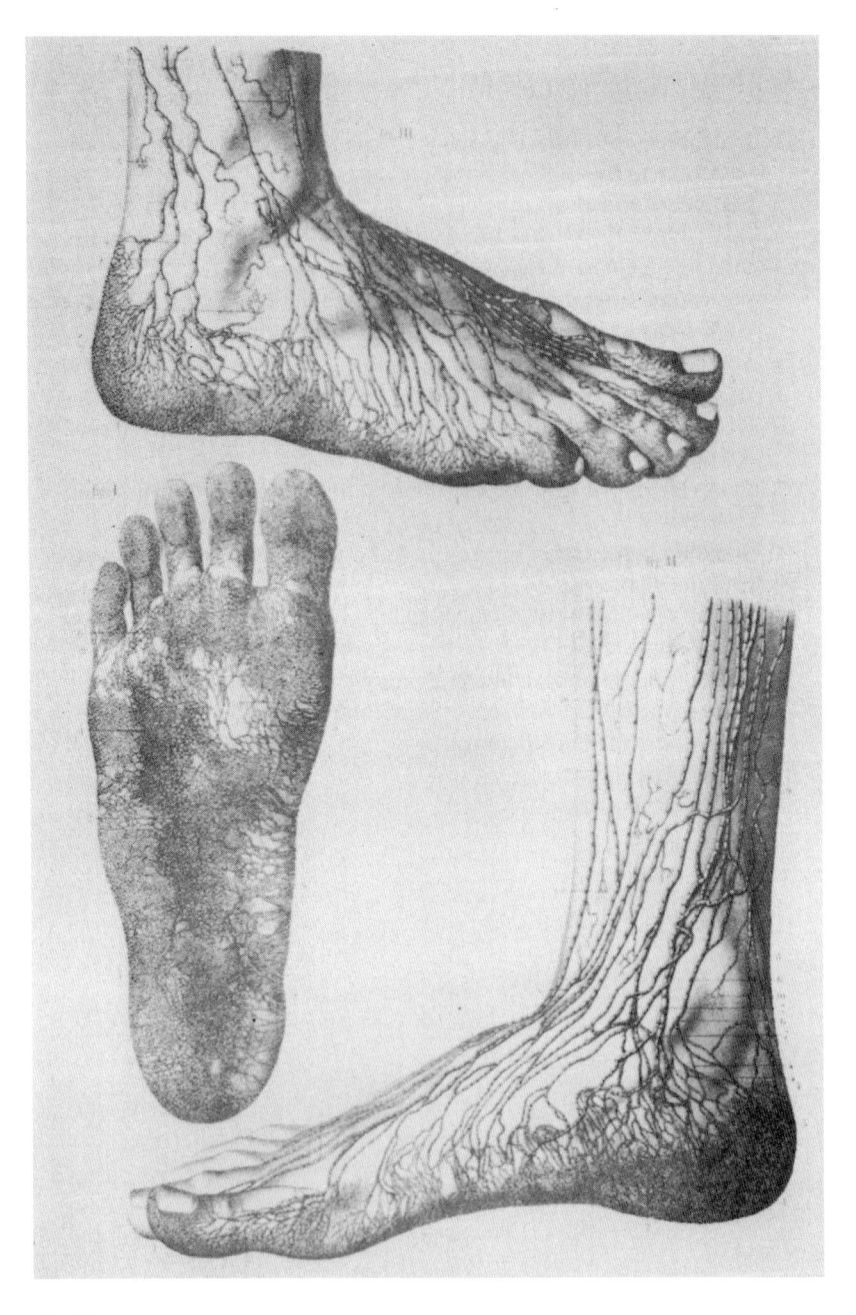

Fig. 13

V Treatment of the nape of the neck (patient prone)

1. Effleurage with rotary technique from the middle of the thoracic vertebrae to the cervical vertebrae. 3 x.

2. Stationary circles over the profundus, middle and terminus. 3 x.

3. Stationary circles below the occiput then middle and terminus. 3 x.

4. Standing behind the patient's head: stationary circles along the nuchal line from the middle of the head to the ears. Treat the entire back of the head in this manner in 3 lines. Each line 3 x.

5. Stationary circles on the side of the head to the terminus. 1 x.

6. Grasp the occiput at the nuchal line, stretch the neck and vibrate. 3 x.

7. Pump technique over the shoulders until the thumbs are in the termini. 3 x.

8. Standing to the left of the neck: Rabbit technique i.e. pump-push over the neck. 3 x.

9. Flat thumb circles in parallel (work on shoulder musculature toward the terminus). 3 x. Flat thumb circles alternating between shoulders. 3 x per shoulder.

10. With 8 fingers in one line, stationary circles on either side of the spine with pressure towards the vertebrae. 3 x.

11. Vibration and final effleurage. 1 x.

1 Massage technique

VI Treatment of the back

1. Effleurage with parallel rotary technique:
   - 3 x movements from the shoulder blades upward.
   - 5 x movements from the midback upward.
   - 7 x movements from the lumbar region upward. 1 x each.
2. Alternating rotary technique over the right shoulder blade and right side of the back. Always start from the spine in a lateral direction in 3 rows down the spine, alternating to the count of six, then 3 rows back up the spine. 3 x.
3. Intercostal spaces with flat fingers using small oval stationary circles. Cover the whole right ribcage. 3 x.
4. Seven technique: beginning with the hand closest to the feet, alternating rotary technique from the spine to the side (count to four) then pump – push without the fingers only along the side to the axilla (count to "se-ven"). 3 x.
5. Large stationary circles in 3 places on the side, working towards the axilla. 3 x.
6. Stationary circles with both hands on the upper arm, two positions on the deltoid (pulling towards you) and one position pushing into the terminus and axilla. 3 x.
7. Change to the other side of the patient and treat the border of the right trapezius using thumb circles. 3 x.
8. Repeat steps 2-7 on the patient's left side.
9. Rotary technique on the extensors of the back: parallel, alternating, and in a number of different rhythmical variations. 3 x each.
10. Triangle between the shoulder blades with flat thumb circles, first parallel 3 x, then alternating to both terminus 3 x each. With 8 fingers make very flat circles, pressure and direction to the right on the right side 3 x, and to the left on the left side 3 x.
11. Edges of the shoulder blade with stationary circles (pads of the fingers) directly over the edges. Pressure always toward the axilla. 3 x.
12. With 8 fingers in one line, stationary circles on either side of the spine with pressure towards the vertebrae. 3 x.
13. Vibration and final effleurage. 1 x.

Sequence of manipulations 1.8

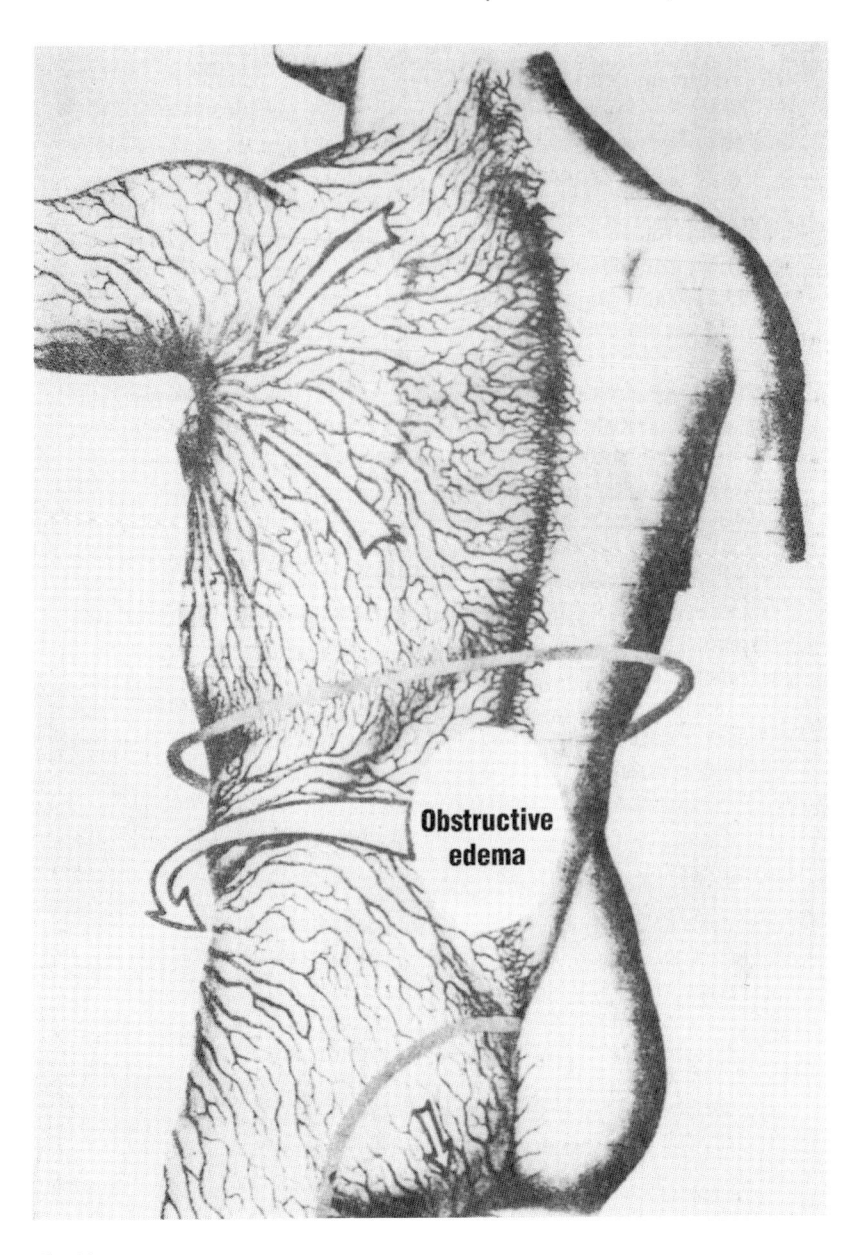

Fig. 14

1 Massage technique

VII Treatment of the buttocks

1. Effleurage with rotary technique, parallel from the sacrum along the lumbar vertebrae. 3 x.
2. Rotary technique parallel, fanning out to the sides (count to seven). The last two motions are circles with flat fingers, no thumbs. 3 x.
3. Rotary technique alternating from the lumbar vertebrae over the right hip and gluteals (buttocks) in 3 rows, 3 x.
4. Stationary circles hand on hand, down and up the iliac crest. Pressure towards the fingertips and circles toward the head. 3 x.
5. Stationary circles below the iliac crest on 3 imaginary semi-circles over the gluteals. Fingers are placed in the direction of lymph flow, pressure towards the fingertips (inguinal lymph nodes) and circles towards the feet. 3 x each semicircle.
6. With 8 fingers in one line, stationary circles on the right side of the lumbar spine and sacrum with pressure towards the vertebrae. 3 x.
7. Stationary circles in 3 places over the quadratus lumborum muscle between the twelfth rib and iliac crest. Pressure inward towards the spine. 3 x.
8. Repeat steps 3-7 on the left side.
9. Sacral triangle with flat thumb circles, parallel 3 x, then alternating in 3 rows on either side 3 x each. Then with 8 fingers flat, as in the shoulder triangle. 3 x.
10. Vibration and final effleurage. 1 x.

Sequence of manipulations 1.8

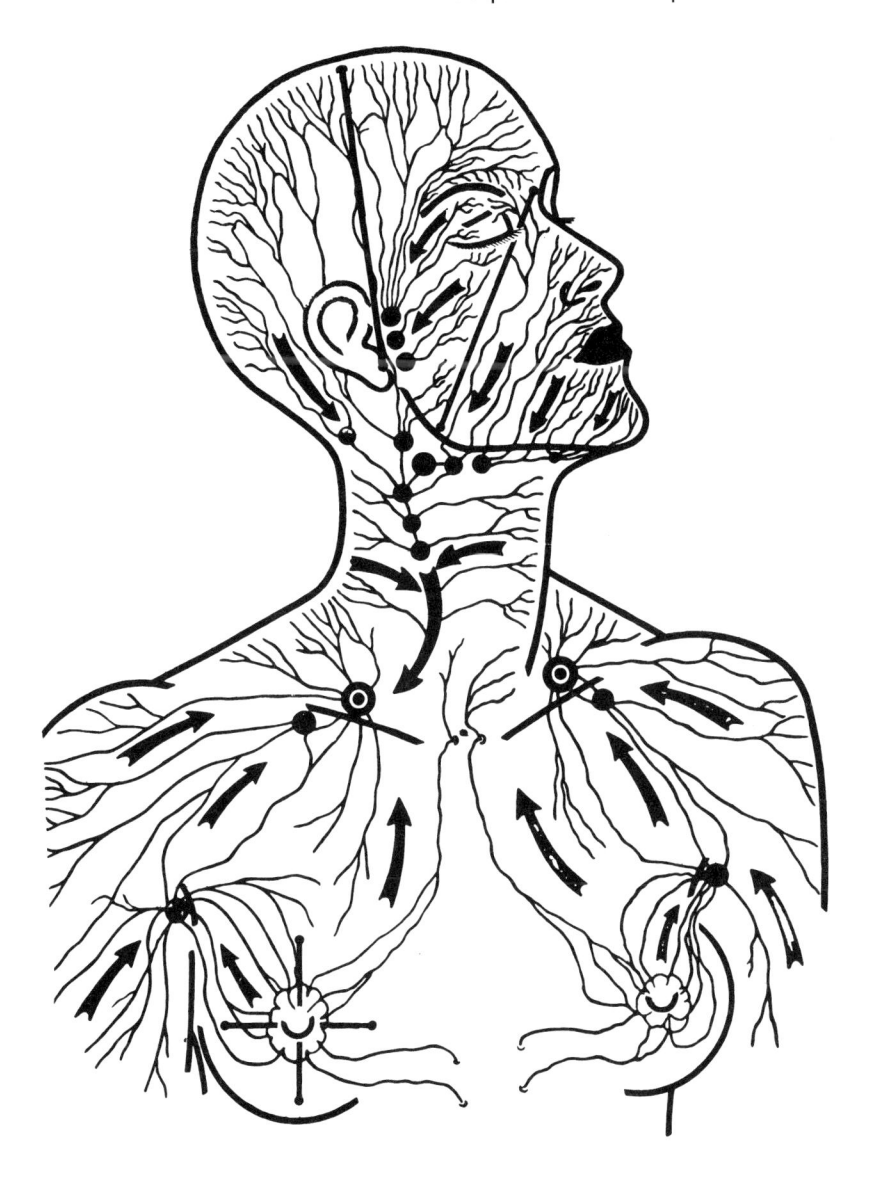

Fig. 15: Schematic representation of lymph drainage from head and neck, breasts (4 quadrants), lymph flow over the shoulder directly to the terminus. (Vodder [1a])

1 Massage technique

VIII Treatment of the chest

1. Rotary technique (effleurage with thumbs) from the sternum to the axilla, parallel motions. 1 x.
2. Stationary circles with flat fingers on the outside of the left breast. If necessary, one hand supports while the other pumps. 3 x.
3. Pump – push along (without thumbs) at the same position. 3 x.
4. Then include the thumbs and using the pump technique below the breast and the rotary above it, drain towards the axilla (pump-push with flat thumb circles). 3 x.
5. Alternating rotary technique over the ribs from the sternum to the side, below the breast. 3 x.
6. Treat the intercostal spaces using small oval circles with the fingers. Pressure inward. 3 x.
7. Origin of the ribs at the sternum with 8 fingers. Pressure into the sternum. 3 x. Then treat the sternum with a flat hand and little pressure. 3 x.
8. 3 large stationary circles with 8 fingers on the side to the axilla. 3 x.
9. Repeat steps 2-8 on the right side.
10. Parallel rotary technique from the sternum towards the sides (count to 4) then parallel finger circles spiraling up towards the axilla (continue to 7). 3 x.
11. Final effleurage. 1 x.

Sequence of manipulations 1.8

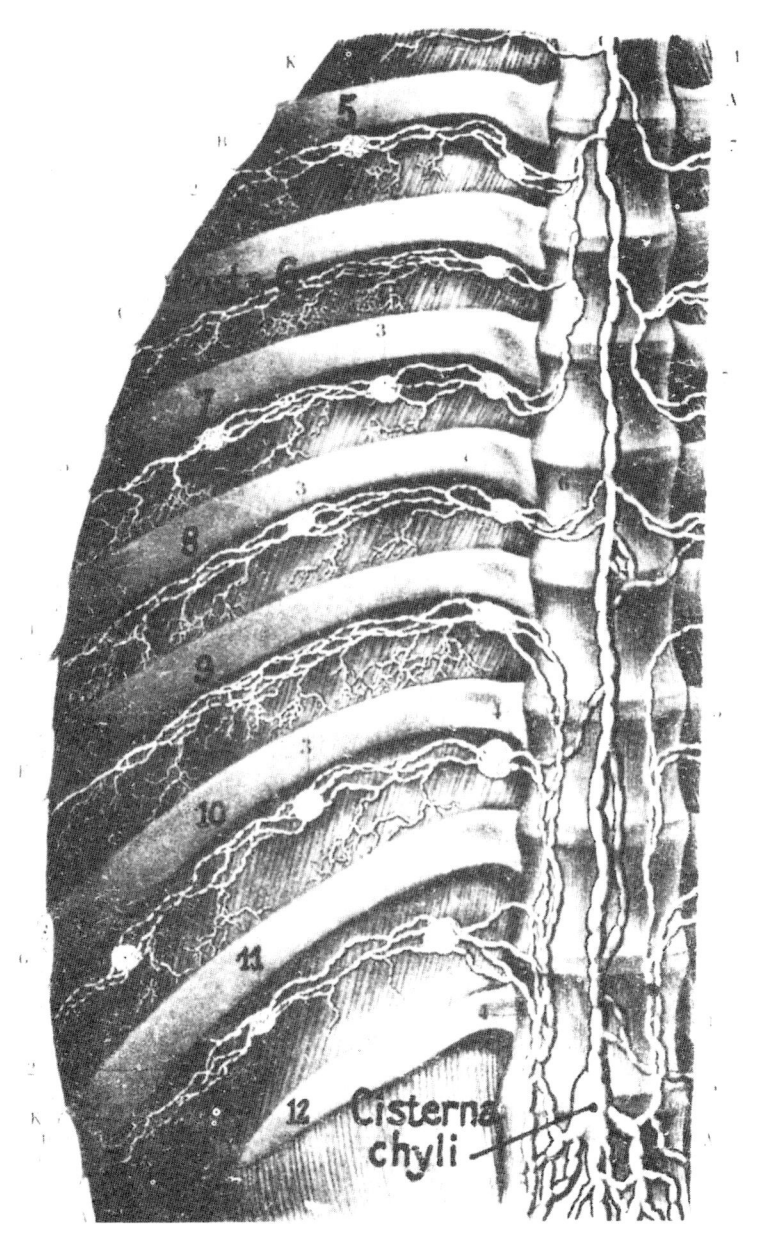

Fig. 16: Beginning of the thoracic duct with the Cisterna chyli. Intercostal lymph pathways and nodes. Truncus lymphaticus descendens dexter et sinister (descending thoracic lymph pathways, Vodder [25])

1 Massage technique

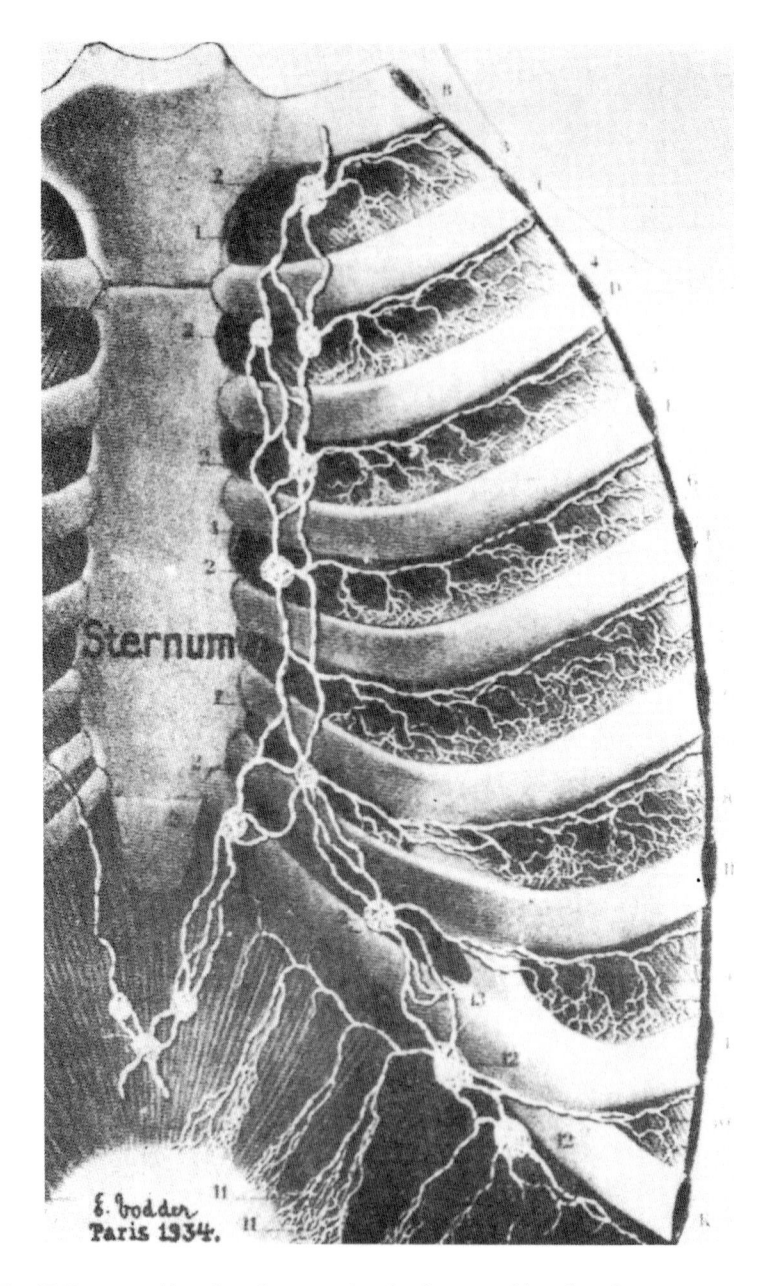

Fig. 17: Parasternal lymph pathways and nodes, intercostal lymph pathways (Vodder [1a])

Sequence of manipulations 1.8

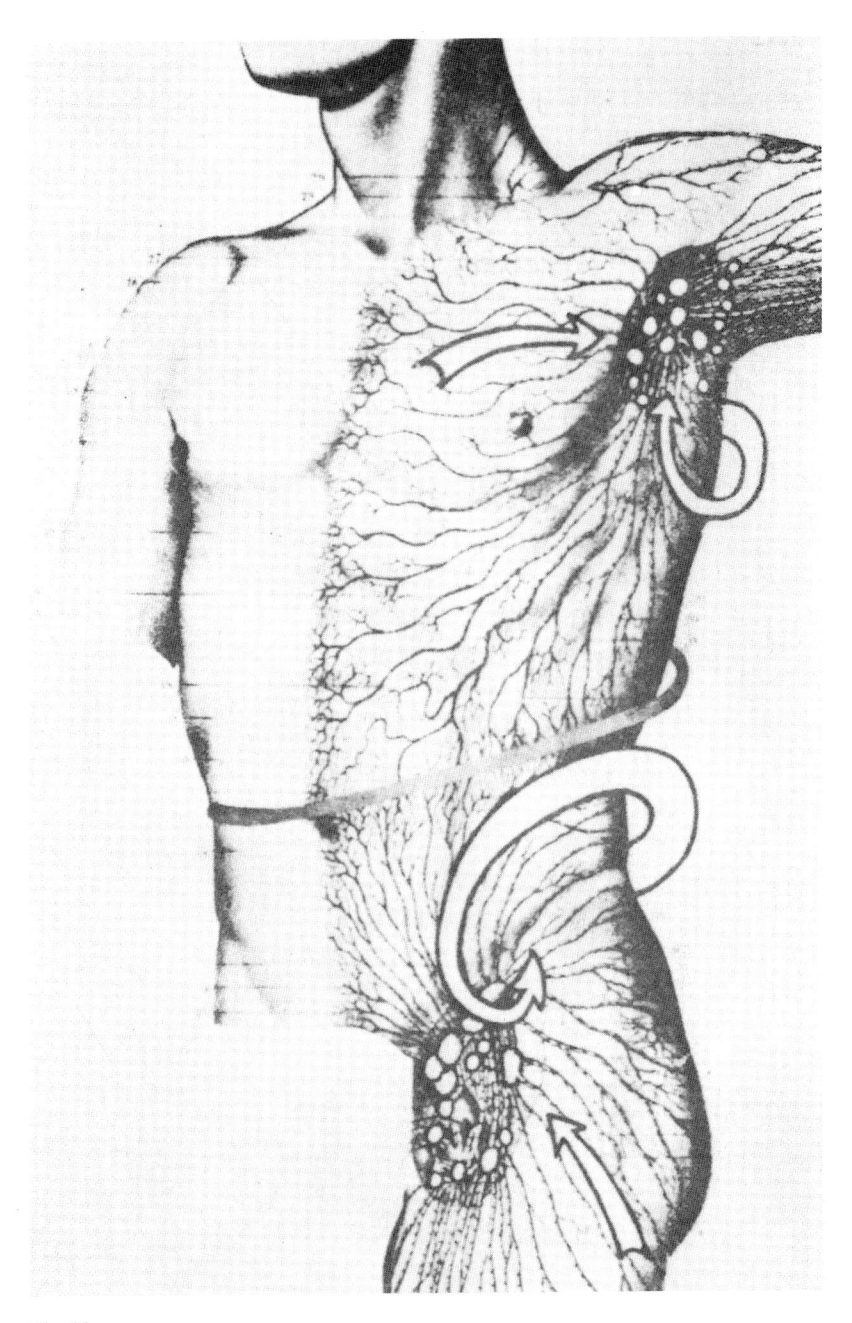

Fig. 18

1 Massage technique

IX Treatment of the abdomen

1. Parallel rotary technique (effleurage) from the pubic bone to below the sternum 1 x, then stroke over the solar plexus with the flat of the hand. 5 x.
2. Stroke over descending colon alternating hands. 5 x.
3. Stroke over descending, ascending then transverse colon using both hands, i.e. in a triangular pattern. 5 x.
4. Treatment of colon: with 4 fingers of one hand on top of 4 fingers of the other, make stationary circles over the descending, ascending, and transverse colon keeping the fingers parallel to the colon. Stretch the skin in the direction of intestinal flow. 3 x.
5. Seven technique: 4 fingers on 4, making progressive circles over the descending colon. Treat the ascending colon with alternating thumb circles, moving towards the hepatic flexure. Then use alternating rotary technique over the transverse colon. Count to "seven" over each part. Repeat 3 x.
6. Weight reduction technique: alternating rotary technique, transversely and if necessary longitudinally over the abdomen. 3 x.
7. Panniculosis technique: small, light skin technique with the thumb twisting the skin against the index finger. 3 lines on either side. Drain from the watershed to the inguinal lymph nodes, paying attention to the direction of drainage in the skin. 3 x each.
8. Treatment of abdominal lymph nodes: deep stationary circles placing 8 fingers above the pubic bone, at the side of the rectus abdominus. Before the pressure phase, the skin is pulled distally with no pressure. Slow movements while looking into the patient's eyes and deep pressure towards the cisterna chyli. 5 x each on each side.
9. Final effleurage with breathing. During inspiration, 3 flat rotary motions from the pubic bone to the sternum. During expiration, parallel stroking with the thumbs along the costal arches then with the fingers along the iliac crests and inguinal ligaments to the pubic bone. 3 x.

X Therapeutic movements – special techniques – oedema therapy

For treating various diseases, skin or tissue changes, we use what is known as therapeutic movements.

These are the same as the techniques described in the practical part of this book. They possess the typical criteria of all manipulations used in lymph drainage: circular movement of the skin with a variation in pressure which is adapted to the symptoms and exerted in the direction of lymph flow. In addition, they are combined with various movements and breathing exercises as well as bandaging if necessary. The duration of treatment is adapted to the symptoms.

Since there are so many indications for MLD and each indication occurs in countless variations, it is impossible to describe therapeutic techniques. They vary from one patient to the next. Training in advanced courses enables the participant to treat any condition for which MLD is indicated. Generally speaking, any part of the body can be adequately treated with the therapeutic movements using typical MLD techniques [27].

2 Dr. Vodder on the technique of Manual Lymph Drainage

[1a] "Working on the lymphatic system in such a way that good therapeutic results are obtained is no easy matter. After all, the lymph vessels are as thin as silk threads and lymph capillaries* are even finer and more delicate. The classical massage techniques have no draining effect. If we massage with hard, stiff movements, we are pressing the blood out of one tissue and into another. The regenerating fluids do not find their own way into the tissue. Sometimes all we achieve is a painful pinching of the capillaries with resulting haematomas. Therefore, we must create a whole new technique.

In order to achieve a movement of water, we have developed a special pumping technique. It is as if a pump draws the fluid and transports it further. In our manual techniques, the hand rotates spirally into and out of the tissue. The lymph-draining action is in the hand and **no** equipment can ever replace an experienced hand. When these refined movements are executed with the consciousness in the fingertips (soft as cat's paws), we produce a calm, relaxed state that promotes lymph flow. Fresh oxygen and active substances penetrate through the interstitial tissue to nourish and regenerate the cells. The circular and spiral drainage manipulations are life-giving movements, as are all spiral oscillations in nature. The hand turning in and out of the tissue with rising and falling pressure (crescendo – decrescendo) is similar to the action of the heart with its systole and diastole.

It is well known that the rhythm of the heart is eight-tenths of a second, during which the heart rests for four-tenths of a second. Thus, the heart rests just as long as it works and in this way can normally operate for a full century without fatigue. We know masseuses who have mastered our method of lymph drainage to such a degree of perfection that they can perform the techniques without fatigue or exertion, delighting in tension and relaxation, building stamina during work renewing energy during the pause. If you work harmoniously you will really feel the flow of natural energy forces; you might call them cosmic forces.

The purpose of lymph drainage is to transport used tissue fluid from the head and various regions of the body to the neck so that new, fresh

---

* The term "lymph capillary" has now been replaced by "initial lymph vessel" -ed.

lymph can flow into the tissues. The drainage must be performed softly, harmoniously, rhythmically, and with supple hands. It is especially important that the wrists remain loose. Hard massage or spasm-like tension can give rise to local constriction of lymph capillaries with the formation of new infiltrations. The hands should be so supple and alive that the dry skin can be massaged. This is especially helpful during examination of the patient."

2.1 Whole body treatment

We would now like to deal with the whole-body treatment. As massage therapists, we are familiar with complete treatments and holistic medical care, even if we are compelled to carry out many partial treatments. We then apologetically say that the reflexes brought about by the treatment do indeed have an impact on the whole person. New massage methods are also developed within these time-saving techniques.

When we carry out whole-body drainage, we are directly influencing 50% of the total connective tissue in the body.

Let us assume that the direct effect of MLD does not penetrate beyond 2 cm below the skin surface. With a skin surface area of 2 square metres and a specific weight of the body of 1.2 (2000 x 2 x 1.2) = 48 kg (105 lbs). Taking the average body weight minus bones, we see that whole-body treatment directly reaches about half of the total body tissue.

In connection with Dr. Vodder's MLD we would also like to mention the Arndt-Schulz biological principle. This says that small or weak stimuli stimulate whereas strong stimuli inhibit or paralyse. To put the effect of MLD in a nutshell:

MLD causes body fluid (connective tissue fluid, lymph and venous blood) to flow, removes waste products from the connective tissue, rectifies metabolic dysfunctions in the interstitium, supports the defence mechanism of the lymph system, balances the nervous system, relieves congestion and satisfies the therapist because she/he can achieve results and help people with a method whose effect can be precisely explained and thus applied selectively.

When Manual Lymph Drainage is combined with other physical therapy methods, any circulatory treatment should be performed before lymph drainage. In treating oedema, bandages of various types, stretch

2 Dr. Vodder on the technique of Manual Lymph Drainage

positions, breathing therapy, a special diet, electrotherapy, and drugs are used. However, Manual Lymph Drainage is and will remain an indispensable part of oedema therapy [34].

APPENDIX

Lymph Drainage – A new therapeutic method serving cosmetic care

First publication about Dr. Vodder's Manual Lymph Drainage, an original work from Dr. Emil Vodder, Paris 1936.

The beauty of the face

A poet describes the eyes as the mirror of the soul. In modern body care, the face could be called the mirror of health. The face not only reflects our feelings of well being and sorrow or our character, but it also reveals our state of health, the balance of mind and body.

The face is also more exposed than the body to the weather, i.e. wind, rain, and temperature changes.

The face also *experiences* more of than the body; it is more *exposed*. Thus in the morning, beauties notice the first signs of transition in their faces, long before the body itself ages. With this shock begins the never ending attempt to maintain beauty and radiance.

Therefore it is not surprising that from time immemorial, we have endeavoured to improve and brighten up the appearance of the face. It also isn't surprising that women who see their youth disappearing spend their time and money to try and stop this. Is it successful? ... That depends on how they invest their time and money.

Yet there are many charlatans with bottomless pockets. Every day incredible sums of money are given away for worthless skin care and beauty products.

Then it is not correct (and we should be clear about this) to cash in on the inadequacies of the face like an ill person who believes he can get rid of his problems by taking tablets. It is just as useless to put a *youth-*cream on a sleepy face. These days, most of the beauty care products are facade cosmetics. In other words, one cannot change the face with surface treatments: peeling of the skin with chemical products, just like smoothing out wrinkles and strengthening the skin with certain cosmetic products are only a trick. Their effect only lasts for a short time because one doesn't get to the root of the problem.

Is aging unavoidable?

If the world continually develops, why can't we also benefit from the advancements? Why is it that we cannot maintain perpetual youth? It is so nice to be young and supple, to shine with beauty and zest for life. Young and healthy people are simply successful in everything. Why therefore does nature allow us to age?

To find the answer we will take an investigative journey through the wondrous world of our bodies.

The blood vessel system

We begin our search in the heart itself, in a small vehicle that we will call a white blood cell. We can examine life more closely in the individual factories along the current in the path formed by our blood vessel network.

At first we are surrounded by numerous smaller boats: the red blood cells which are loaded with oxygen, the fuel for all cell activity. The water in our current is called plasma and is yellow: it contains nutrients and wastes. Each heartbeat sends our small vehicle, in the incredible time of 23 seconds, through the whole blood vessel system (arteries, capillaries and veins) until it has reached the heart again.

The lymph vessel system

Until now this was really unknown to the general public because circulation always referred to the blood circulation.

A new system? Absolutely not, as the lymph system is the origin of life, the lymph* is the nutrient liquid for the very first collection of cells just as it is for the living palace of millions of cells – the complete human organism.

However this system was discovered relatively late: there are two noteworthy 17th century scholars of the lymph system: Pecquet (1647) who discovered and named the cisterna chyli and the Dane, Bartholin who discovered the lymph vessel system three years later.

Thus we live in lymph*, i.e. our tissues are washed in lymph*. It supplies us with the life giving nutrients necessary for body development.

If we continue on our journey, we see how youth, life and death are dependent on lymph and its renewal.

Our vehicle has now left the capillaries through a small secret door and in this manner we can distinguish between the two circulatory systems.

Lymph is a whitish fluid. The flow in the lymph channels is sluggish and we glide calmly through because there is no pulsation here coming from the heart and driving us forward every few seconds. However we still move forward with the help of a carefully thought out valve system that prevents backflow: We pass thousands of filters until we reach the large lakes of the serous cavities. In this way we can visit all regions of the body from head to feet, e.g. the labyrinth of the ear, the membranes of the brain and spinal cord, the pleura etc. We run into flooded regions (oedema and infiltrations) and dry areas where life functions slower and cells degenerate because the lymph* was the source of their renewal.

The lymph vessel system therefore represents a type of sewage system, eliminating wastes produced by the working cells and carrying them to organs which get rid of them – the lymph nodes.

The lymph nodes

We are concerned here with filters, whose function is to hold back and destroy the harmful substances, poisons and bacteria. A lymph node consists of adenoid tissue and continually produces white blood cells, like the spleen and tonsils. These cells defend the body against invasion and poisoning and their activity is heightened during infectious diseases. So what happens in the lymph system during an infection (e.g. during a heavy cold)? We experience a battle. The body reacts to the invasion of bacteria in the nose with an immediate assembly of troops, a total security force. The mucous membranes swell up, the lymph vessels

---

* As this article was written, all bodily fluid excepting blood and cellular fluid was described as *lymph*. Now this is referred to in the nomenclature as *connective tissue fluid*.

and nodes enlarge, the white blood cells destroy bacteria and take them away. Generally the battle is finished in the lymph nodes, which can be compared to castles. It is fascinating to watch this process under the microscope and it gave rise to Claude Bernard's conclusion: "Bacteria themselves are not the decisive factor, solely the surrounding territory".

We should be clear that a poor functioning lymph circulation lowers our defence which opens the door to every infection such as catarrh, chronic colds, sinusitis, sore throat, angina etc. Unfortunately, this condition of congestion which can be traced back to a worsening and stagnation of lymph, also has a detrimental effect on one's appearance. This is the deeper cause of a series of cosmetic flaws such as swelling, reddening, puffiness, bags under the eyes, pimples, couperose, etc.

Stagnation of the lymph flow, therefore has catastrophic results for health and beauty: one must get the lymph circulation going again at all costs and this is achieved with the help of Manual Lymph Drainage. MLD cleanses the lymph*, the swelling in the mucous membranes goes down and consequently the cause of the problems is eradicated.

The natural regeneration of skin through lymph drainage

Before we go back to the heart, we conclude our investigative journey by examining the skin. We see that the skin cells wear out and thanks to a process called mitosis, are constantly replaced by young cells.

We have seen how the necessary, life-sustaining nutrients leave the blood with the help of osmosis, pass into the lymph* and thus reach the cells. Assuming this exchange cannot take place, the lymph vessels become blocked with stagnant, old lymph. The blood flows, to no avail, past each little *secret door* and transports the nutrients to another location. This is how the body becomes poisoned by its own wastes.

During my research work in the laboratories of the faculty in Copenhagen (1922-24), under the direction of the renowned cancer researcher Prof. Fibiger, the significance of the cell environment in lymph circulation for living, diseased, and dead cells was suddenly clear to me. I understood clearly how the perpetual youth of the cell depends on this fluid (the lymph*).

Dr. Carrel's experiments have supported my theories. He was able to keep embryonic cells alive for over 10 years, whereas the normal life expectancy is only 4–5 years. This was possible thanks to the lymphatic* milieu which was changed every 2 days.

Conclusion: If the milieu and cell activity stagnate then the cells will degenerate, age and die. If the milieu is constantly renewed then life flourishes and the cells divide. Then the wrinkled and tired skin can regenerate itself, it becomes fresh and elastic and the tired worn-out appearance in the face disappears. A real metamorphosis is experienced, a natural regeneration that comes from within.

Our new therapeutic method is therefore based on these facts.

Lymph drainage

After many years of clinical experience and research, a rational method of treatment has been successfully developed which enables renewal of the lymph*, activation of the circulation, stimulation of cell activity and regeneration of the facial tissue.

Lymph drainage is a healthy, natural, painless and absolutely effective method which gives a new basis to life, health and beauty.

Original translation into German by Mechtild Yvon, M.A. Phil. of Vienna.

We thank Mrs. Banniza of Menden for her great effort in procuring this article.

Nothing is added to this article. The special thing about it is that it was written 60 years ago. Vodder's ideas of that time were proved correct through experiments in many ways. His manual techniques need no improvement or further development. The method only needs further research of its actions. This is the task before us today and, at the same time, a legacy left to us.

Bibliography

[1] *Vodder, E.:* Le drainage lymphatique, une nouvelle méthode thérapeutique. Santé pour tous, 1936.
[1a] *Vodder, E.:* Die manuelle Lymphdrainage ad modum Vodder. Instruktionsheft mit Behandlungstafeln (1970).
[2] *Helmrich, H.E.:* Muskelverspannungen als Krankheit. Erfahrungsheilkunde 26/12 (1977) 605-614.
–: Muskelverspannung als Krankheit. Schriftenreihe Erfahrungsheilkunde. Bd. 20. Karl F. Haug, Heidelberg 2. Aufl. 1984.
[3] *Kuhnke, E.:* Der Schmerz als Reflex, Empfindung und Affekt. Physiotherapie 65/4.
[4] *Kownatzki, E.:* Antigene und Antigenität. Aus: *Vorlaender, K.O.:* Praxis der Immunologie. Thieme, Stuttgart 1976.
[5] *Vorlaender, K.O.:* Vortrag bei der 8. wissenschaftlichen Arbeitstagung der Ges. f. Man. Lymphdrainage nach Dr. Vodder (1975).
[6] *Hahn, H./Opferkuch, W.:* Mechanismen der immunologischen Infektabwehr. Aus: *Vorlaender, K.O:* Praxis der Immunologie. Thieme, Stuttgart 1976.
[7] *Wendt, L.:* Krankheiten verminderter Kapillarmembranpermeabilität. E. Koch, 1973.
[8] *Resch, K.:* Zelluläre Immunreaktionen. Aus: *Vorlaender, K.O.:* Praxis der Immunologie. Thieme, Stuttgart 1976.
[9] *Mislin, H.:* Handbuch der allgemeinen Pathologie. 3. Bd., 6. Teil, Springer, Heidelberg/New York 1972.
[9a] *Pischinger, A.:* Das System der Grundregulation. Karl F. Haug, Heidelberg 9. Aufl. 1998.
[10] *Babor, M.:* Vortrag beim Fortbildungstag der Ges. f. Manuelle Lymphdrainage nach Dr. Vodder in Walchsee, am 3.4.1976.
[11] *Casley-Smith, J. R.:* Electron microscopical observations on the dilated Lymphathics in oede-mateous regions and their sollaps following Hyaluronidase administration. Brit. J. Exp. Path. 48 (1967) 680-689.
[12] *Mislin, H.:* Vortrag bei der wissenschaftlichen Arbeitstagung der Ges. f. Man. Lymphdrainage nach Dr. Vodder, Hamburg 1973.
[13] *Földi, M.:* Handbuch der allgemeinen Pathologie. 3. Bd., 6. Teil. Springer, Heidelberg/New York 1972.
[14] *Kuhnke, E.:* Prinzipien des Stofftransportes im Organismus. Physiotherapie 64/1.
[15] *Börcsök, E/Földi, K./Földi, M./Wittlinger, G.:* Zur therapeutischen Beeinflussung des akuten experimentellen lymphostatischen Ödems mit Vitaminen, vitaminartigen Stoffen sowie mittels Massage. Angiologica 8/31 (1971).
[16] *Földi-Börcsök, E./Casley-Smith, J.R./Földi, M.:* The treatment of experimental Lymphoedema. Angiologica 9 (1972) 92-98.
[17] *Stewart, P.B:* The rate of formation and lymphatic removal of fluid in pleural effusions. J. Clinic Invest. 42 (1963) 258-262.
[18] *Földi, M.:* Erkrankungen des Lymphsystems. Witzstrock, Baden-Baden/Brüssel 1977.
[19] *Price, E.W.:* Endemic elephantiasis of lower legs in Ethiopia. Abstract: III. Int. Congr. Lymphologie, Brüssel 1970, p. 71.
[20] *Földi, M./Simon, M./Schneider, J./Börcsök, E./Maurer, M./Lehotal, L.:* Characteristic striation and ridge pattern of the cervical skin in Lymphogenic encephalopathy. Acta paediat. Acad. Sci. hung. 9 (1967) 262-272.
[21] *Wendt, L.:* Immunologie auf neuen Wegen. E. Koch, 1975.
[22] *Wendt, L.:* Vortrag bei den 2. Fortbildungstagen des Ges. f. Manuelle Lymphdrainage nach Dr. Vodder, Baden-Baden 1980.
[23] *Tischendorf, F.:* Zur funktionellen Grob- und Feinstruktur des lymphatischen Systems. Sonderdruck Nr. 49/51/52, 9.12.1977, Schattauer.

Bibliography

[24] *Wendt, L./Wendt, Th.:* Gibt es einen physiologischen Eiweißspeicher des Menschen? Erfahrungsheilkunde 10 (1980) 805-819.
[25] *Tischendorf, F.:* Lymphatisches System. Demeter, 1980.
[26] *Marnitz, H.:* Ungenutzte Wege der manuellen Behandlung. Karl F. Haug, Heidelberg 1981.
[27] *Vodder, E.:* Die technische Grundlage der manuellen Lymphdrainage. Physikalische Therapie 1 (1983) 17.
[28] *Tischendorf, F.:* Persönliche Mitteilung 1983.
[29] *Mislin, H.:* Die Lymphdrainage als biotechnisches Problem. Vortrag bei den 3. Fortbildungstagen der Ges. f. Manuelle Lymphdrainage nach Dr. Vodder in Baden-Baden, 1982.
[30] *Seeger, P.G.:* Leitfaden für Krebsleidende und die es nicht werden wollen. Mehr Wissen, Düsseldorf 1982, p. 77/78/89.
[31] *Kubik, St.:* Drainagemöglichkeiten der Lymphterritorien nach Verletzungen peripherer Kollektoren und nach Lymphadenektomie. Folia Angiologica Vol. XXVIII, p. 7/8/9/80.
[32] *Brunner, U.:* Das Lymphödem der unteren Extremität. Hans Huber, Bern 1961.
[33] *Vester, F.:* Phänomen Streß. Dtv, München 1981.
[34] *Wittlinger, Gebh.:* Die Wertigkeit der Manuellen Lymphdrainage bei der Behandlung von lymphostatischen Ödemen. Physikalische Therapie 4/9 (1983) 447-448.
[35] *Hecht, L.:* Orthopädie, Rheumatologie, Unfallchirurgie, Perimed, p. 37-39.
[36] *Partilla, W.:* Erfahrungsheilkunde 29/4 (1980). Karl F. Haug, Heidelberg.
[37] *Reitter, K.:* Indikationsliste für die Fachpresse. Ges. f. Manuelle Lymphdrainage nach Dr. Vodder.
[38] Acta lymphologica 1 (1979). Verlag für Medizin Dr. Ewald Fischer, Heidelberg.
[39] Acta lymphologica 2/3 (1980/81). Verlag für Medizin Dr. Ewald Fischer, Heidelberg.
[40] Erfahrungsheilkunde 33/9 (1984). Karl F. Haug, Heidelberg.
[41] *Földi E./Földi, M./Tischendorf, F.:* Adipositas, Lipödem und Lymphostase. Die Medizinische Welt (1983) 198-200, Schattauer.
[42] *Funes, J.F./Funes, L.N.:* Cirugia Plastica con Tratamiento pre y post operatorio de drenaje linfatico manual. Vortrag beim 7. Congresco National de Estetica, Cosmetologia S. – 7. 2. 1984 in Mexico City.
[43] *Földi/Tischendorf:* Lipödem und Zellulitis. Medizinischer Verlag Erdmann-Prenger, München 1985.
[44] Kosmetik international 1 (1987).
[45] *Curri, S.B.:* Schriftenreihe "Manuelle Lymphdrainage nach Dr. Vodder" – Referate. Karl F. Haug, Heidelberg 1984.
[46] *Curri, S.B.:* Schriftenreihe "Manuelle Lymphdrainage nach Dr. Vodder" – Ödem, Lymphödem und perivaskulare Grundsubstanz. Eine klinische Studie über die sog. Zellulitis. Karl F. Haug, Heidelberg 1988.
[47] *Kubik, St./Manestar, M.:* Anatomie der Lymphkapillaren und Präkollektoren der Haut. In: *Bonninger, A./Partsch, H.:* Initiale Lymphstrombahn. Internat. Symposium Zürich 1984. G. Thieme, Stuttgart/New York 1984, p. 62-69.
[48] *Hutzschenreuter, P./Brümmer, H.:* Die Wirkung der Lymphdrainage auf die Vasomotion. Lymphol. (1988).